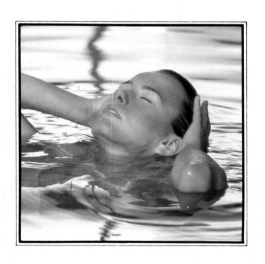

UK Price
£3.95

A FAMILY GUIDE TO HEALTHY LIVING
COPING WITH
STRESS

DR TOM TRAUER

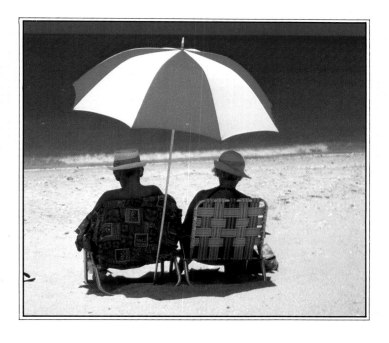

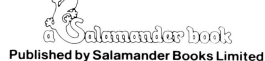
a Salamander book

Published by Salamander Books Limited
LONDON • NEW YORK

A SALAMANDER BOOK

Acknowledgements
The author and publisher would like to thank the following for permission
to quote excerpts from published material:

C.L. Cooper, *The Stress Check*, Prentice Hall, 1981, for the Job Stress
questionnaire on page 49.
T. Holmes and R. Rahe, 'The Social Readjustment Rating Scale' published
in the *Journal of Psychosomatic Research*, vol II, 1967, for the Life Events
scale on pages 14-15.
Charles Spielberger, *Understanding Stress and Anxiety*, Harper and
Row, 1979, for the Text Anxiety questionnaire on page 44.

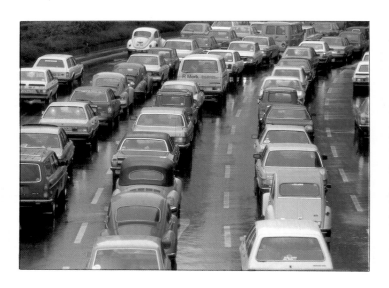

Editor: John Woodward
Designer: Kathy Gummer
Colour reproductions:
Melbourne Graphics

Filmset: Chelmsford Origination
Printed in Belgium by
Proost International Book
Production, Turnhout

AUTHOR

Dr Tom Trauer graduated in psychology at the University of Melbourne, Australia. He trained in clinical psychology and worked for some years in psychiatric hospitals in Melbourne before moving to the UK in 1970. After completing his PhD. at St George's Hospital, London in 1974 he worked for six years at Guy's Hospital, and is now head of the clinical psychology department at King's College Hospital, London. He has a wide range of research interests, and has written numerous articles concerning the 'therapeutic community' movement. His main clinical interest is the effects of brain damage, and he is actively engaged in training clinical psychologists.

CONTENTS

INTRODUCTION

Stress is a commonly used word in the English language, and we all have some idea of what it means. Most people will probably think of it as an unpleasant state of mind brought on by situations which they find difficult to handle. It has something to do with feeling anxious, tense, worried and under strain. It is the opposite of feeling calm and relaxed.

As a starting point to getting a better understanding of stress, it is useful to think of the way engineers or builders use the words stress and strain. For example, a weight resting on a wooden plank places the plank under *stress*. If the weight is heavy enough, the wood in the plank is distorted or compressed. These internal forces within the material of the plank ˜re known as *strain*. If the weight is too heavy for the plank it may become permanently bent, or it may even break ('stress fracture').

If you now think of a person instead of a wooden plank, you can imagine that a stressful event, such as losing a job or having to have an operation, would lead to certain strain reactions within that person, such as tension or worry. It is usually these internal reactions to unpleasant experiences — the strain caused by the stressful situation — that people describe as 'stress'.

This simple model is fine as far as it goes, but it cannot explain certain facts about human stress. For one thing, not everyone regards the same events or experiences as stressful. Some people become very worried and fearful if they have to take a flight in an aeroplane, but other people positively enjoy it. There is evidence that even after major natural disasters like earthquakes, which most of us would think of as very stressful, up to a quarter of the population carry on fairly normally, and show none of the usual signs of stress. What is stressful for one person is not always stressful for another.

Another awkward fact which the simple engineering model cannot

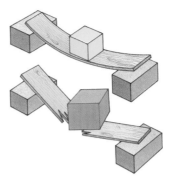

Above: *A simple model of stress. A weight, or stress, creates a strain in the plank, which bends (top). More weight equals more stress: the plank is overstrained and breaks. But people are not planks ...*

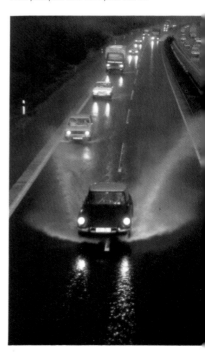

Above: *The problems created by bad driving conditions are similar for every driver on the road, but the reactions of each individual may be very different.*

8

explain is that some people seek out frightening or dangerous activities for fun or recreation. An example of this is parachute jumping. Research has shown that soldiers who are about to jump show many of the common stress signs, such as a fast heartbeat and high levels of adrenalin in the bloodstream, and many of them experience fear. These reactions can be so intense that some soldiers cannot complete their parachute training. But we also know that some people enjoy these same reactions, and consider them part of the thrill of the whole experience.

It seems, therefore, that we need to perceive or judge a situation as harmful or dangerous before we respond with anxiety, tension or worry. The process looks something like this:

DANGER▷PERCEPTION▷ANXIETY
OF DANGER

It is obvious that people have very different ideas when it comes to assessing dangerous situations, and this is why stress means something different to each of us.

Stress, then, is not simply caused by the demands placed upon us by our environment; nor is it solely a symptom of failings in our physical or psychological constitutions. It has to do with our evaluation of the balance between the real or perceived demands placed upon us, and our real or perceived capacity for dealing with those demands. When we judge that the demands exceed our capacities we

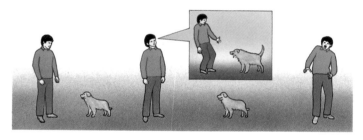

Above: *The degree of anxiety we experience in any situation does not depend on the real threat involved, but on the threat we believe to be involved. A man who believes all dogs are vicious will assume that any strange dog will attack him, and will react with fear and avoidance—regardless of the dog's actual behaviour.*

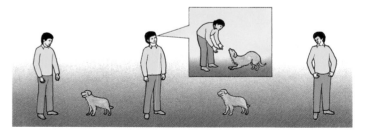

Above: *In contrast, a man who believes all dogs are tame and friendly will assume the same of a strange dog, and will remain quite unconcerned. (Of course, he may be wrong, and the apparently friendly dog may bite him.) In both cases the actual situation is the same: only the man's interpretation of it is different.*

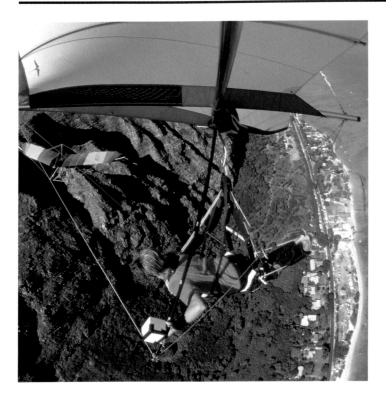

may experience what we call 'stress' (or fear or depression or something similar). Our behaviour will change as a result, and certain changes will occur in the way our bodies function. These alterations in our experience, behaviour and body functions will 'feed back', affecting our perception of the imbalance between external demands and internal capacities. This may aggravate the total stress reaction, or it may reduce it.

Stress and coping

How well we cope with stress will depend upon a number of factors. First of all there is evidence that there are inborn differences between people in their vulnerability to stress: some are more prone to problems than others. Secondly, familiarity with certain stressful events will enable an individual to cope better with them. Thirdly,

Above: *Hang gliding is a dangerous, demanding activity, which you would expect to be stressful — but people do it for fun.*

accurate and relevant knowledge about the real dangers of some worrying future event, like a surgical operation, is always helpful. In particular it can prevent people exaggerating real dangers and imagining unreal dangers. Fourthly, situations are generally less stressful if we have a measure of control over them. Learning how to control our reactions in situations we previously regarded as uncontrollable can be very stress-reducing. Lastly, the role of personal and social support, both in childhood and in adulthood, must not be underestimated. It is easier to cope with stressful events and the reactions they lead to if you have the support of others.

DO YOU SUFFER FROM STRESS?		
Behavioural signs		
Do you smoke?	YES	NO
Do you have problems sleeping?	YES	NO
Do you often get minor illnesses, like colds and flu?	YES	NO
Do you overeat?	YES	NO
Do you consume more alcohol than is good for you?	YES	NO
Have you had much time away from work?	YES	NO
Emotional signs		
Do you worry excessively?	YES	NO
Are you short tempered?	YES	NO
Do you find it hard to concentrate?	YES	NO
Do you often feel anxious or fearful?	YES	NO
Are you excessively concerned about your physical health?	YES	NO
Have you lost your sense of humour?	YES	NO
Physical signs		
Do you notice your heart racing?	YES	NO
Do you often get headaches?	YES	NO
Do you sometimes feel breathless or faint?	YES	NO
Do you sometimes feel hot and sweaty?	YES	NO
Do you often get indigestion or diarrhoea?	YES	NO
Do you often get a dry mouth?	YES	NO
The more questions you answered 'yes' to, the more likely you are to have a stress problem—although you may have been unaware of it.		

INGREDIENTS OF STRESS ═══

Despite the fact that we all find different events and situations stressful, it is possible to list certain situations which are stressful for practically everyone. First among these are occasions where there is a real threat of death or physical injury. Prehistoric man must have found the everpresent danger of man-eating animals threatening and stressful. In fact, his ability to experience fear in the presence of a lion would have had a positive survival value for him—it would have enabled him to take the appropriate action: either 'flight' or 'fight'.

Modern man rarely encounters lions, but there is nevertheless no shortage of dangerous, life-threatening things in our environment. House fires and road traffic accidents are a threat to us all, and some people develop physical and psychological stress reactions as a consequence. Studies of the survivors of fires show that there is a more or less natural sequence of recovery from the stress of the event. First there is the initial shock. Then the person comes to terms with the consequences of the disaster, which may be personal injury, or the death or injury of relatives or friends. Only after these stages have been gone through does the final recovery occur. When formerly well-adjusted people experience difficulties in working their way through this process, it is rarely because of the terror or horror of the event itself. Usually it is something to do with problems in personal and social relationships, such as conflict or guilt if relatives or close friends have been injured or died in the same disaster.

Invasive medical techniques

Below: *To the apprehensive patient, the prospect of surgery can be almost as terrifying as an actual threat to life.*

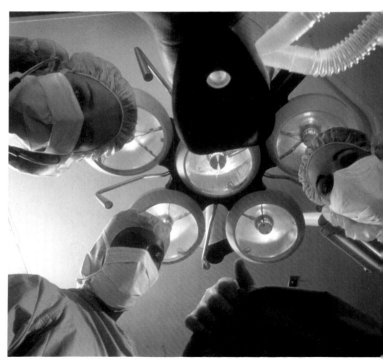

such as surgical operations and certain dental procedures are commonly regarded as very stressful. Researchers investigating this have shown that there are three main ways in which surgical patients anticipate their operations. Some become highly apprehensive, fearful and anxious in the period leading up to the operation. Others are moderately fearful and appropriately worried, whilst a third group are calm, placid and seemingly 'ideal' patients.

It is the second group which tends to do best emotionally after the operation. Patients in the highly anxious group often experience anxiety long after their operation, and the calm and placid individuals often suffer from disturbance, afterwards, in the form of anxiety,

Below: *Chronic stress, although comparatively undramatic, can be more destructive than acute panic in the long term.*

apprehension, anger, hostility or irritability. This evidence suggests that both over-reacting, by panic and excessive worry, and under-reacting by being unnaturally calm and detached, are less effective ways of coping with a common source of stress than an intermediate 'realistic' response.

Of course, not all sources of stress are as dramatic or obvious as disasters and operations. Threats to our personal and social relationships, like the death or emigration of close friends, bereavement and divorce can be very powerful stressors. So can threats to our sense of worth and our good opinion of ourselves. Many people will think worse of themselves on account of examination failure, loss of a job, arrest or imprisonment. The following section looks at a very wide range of personal experiences which have been found to be sources of stress.

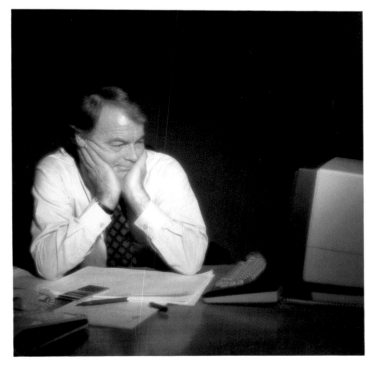

We have known for a long time that adverse events in one's life can herald the onset of an illness, or can make an existing condition worse. In 1967 two American researchers, Thomas Holmes and Richard Rahe, produced a scale called the Social Readjustment Rating Scale (SRRS) designed to measure the amount of disruption caused by such life changes. They asked thousands of subjects to rate how much behavioural readjustment would be needed to cope with a variety of life events, using marriage as a basis for comparison. A very high level of agreement was achieved between the participants for the 43 events which comprise the scale (see below). Each event has a value in Life Change Units which represents the degree of readjustment which it would entail, compared to marriage which is given a value of 50. It can

Life events	Life change units
Death of spouse	100
Divorce	73
Marital separation	65
Jail term	63
Death of close family member	63
Personal injury or illness	53
Marriage	50
Fired at work	47
Marital reconciliation	45
Retirement	45
Change in health of family member	44
Pregnancy	40
Sex difficulties	39
Gain of new family member	39
Business readjustment	39
Change in financial state	38
Death of close friend	37
Change to a different line of work	36
Change in number of arguments with spouse	35
Taking on a large mortgage	31
Foreclosure of mortgage or loan	30

be seen that whilst most of the events are unpleasant, not all of them are. Promotion, outstanding personal achievement and holidays also require adapting to.

The SRRS has been used to explore the relationship between life changes and illness. Holmes and Rahe found that the two years prior to the onset of an illness were often marked by a cluster of life events. They found that, for Americans, there was an increased risk of a serious illness if a total of 300 or more Life Change Units were obtained by an individual over a two-year period.

Later research on negative life events, especially those at the top of the list, shows that the effect of such changes varies considerably depending on the individual's own ability to cope and the availability of social support and help.

Life events	Life change units
Change in responsibility at work	29
Son or daughter leaving home	29
Trouble with in-laws	29
Outstanding personal achievement	28
Wife begins or stops work	26
Children begin or end school	26
Change in living conditions	25
Revision of personal habits	24
Trouble with boss	23
Change in work hours or conditions	20
Change in residence	20
Change in schools	20
Change in recreation patterns	19
Change in social activities	18
Taking on a small mortgage or loan	17
Change in sleeping habits	16
Change in number of family get-togethers	15
Change in eating habits	15
Holiday	13
Christmas	12
Minor violations of the law	11

In order to understand fully our own experience of stress we need to know something about the nature of emotions. It has been known for a very long time that there is a close connection between external events, body reactions and emotions, although there has been debate over just how they are linked. The first scientific theory explaining their interrelationship was put forward by James and Lange 100 years ago. They proposed that when the brain received and analyzed information about the environment, messages were sent through the nerve pathways causing characteristic physical reactions. Our emotional experience was then determined by our perception of these bodily changes. Thus, in contrast to the common-sense view that 'We run because we are afraid' James and Lange were suggesting that 'We are afraid because we run'. This idea is not as peculiar as it sounds when one considers the remark of a trainee parachute jumper: 'I was not afraid at all, until I looked down and

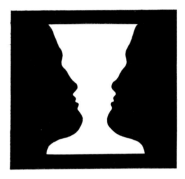

Above: *This drawing can be seen as either a vase or two faces, depending on whether you assume the background is black or white. In the same way emotional reactions to events can alter with changed assumptions. Right: The James-Lange theory suggested that feelings of fear or excitement were stimulated by body changes. In the Cannon theory emotional and physical reactions stem from the thalamus.* Below: *A classic stress situation — parachutists preparing to jump.*

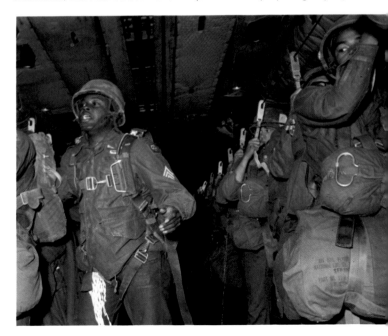

JAMES-LANGE THEORY   CANNON THEORY

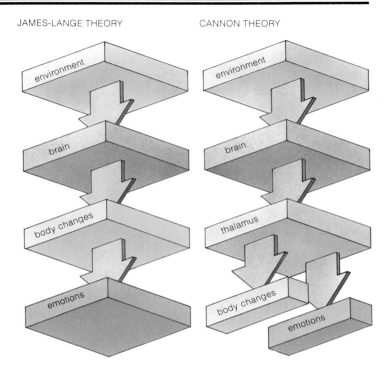

saw my knees trembling. Then I realized how scared I really was'.

This theory remained popular for many years because it was the only one which systematically connected physiology and psychology. It was in the late 1920s, after considerable advances in both subjects, that the theory was superseded by one which fitted the evidence better. This was the theory of a man named Cannon who proposed that when external information reached the brain, it was analyzed unconsciously and relayed to an important brain centre known as the thalamus. The thalamus then did two things: it sent messages to body organs such as the heart, altering their activity levels, and it relayed messages back to the conscious part of the brain which were experienced as emotions. Although Cannon was mistaken about the precise function of the thalamus, his basic theory is still considered to be right.

The important role of the brain in the production of an emotional response is the *appraisal* of the incoming sensory information. Perception and appraisal is not a simple matter of registering external events as a camera or a tape recorder does. The brain *interprets* and *makes sense of* the messages it receives from the sensory organs.

Our perceptions are strongly determined by the assumptions we make about the environment. For example, the drawing on page 16 may be seen as either a vase or as two faces in profile depending on whether you assume that the dark or the light areas are the background. Normally the assumptions we make about our environment depend upon our logical expectations, and also our needs. The effect of needs upon perception can be observed from the way a starving person is likely to hallucinate about food, and thirsty travellers in the desert will

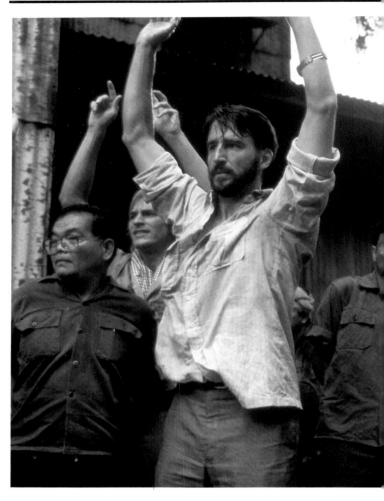

'perceive' the heat haze mirage on the horizon as water.

The way in which our evaluation of a situation can determine our emotional response was clearly shown in an interesting experiment. Four groups of (male) subjects were shown a film of an Australian aboriginal circumcision ceremony. For one group there was no sound-track provided. For the second group the sound-track was a detached, unemotional commentary on the circumcision procedure. The sound-track that the third group heard minimized the unpleasant and painful aspects while stressing the positive features of the ritual. The sound-track for the fourth group emphasized the pain and suffering involved.

Each subject's physiological stress response (the sweat response) was measured throughout the screening, and clear differences emerged between the four groups although they all saw the same film. The sound-track affected the appraisal of what was seen: those subjects who heard the disturbing sound-track had a strong stress response. Those who heard

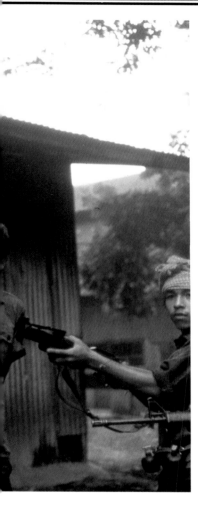

decreased stress responses.

The role of the mind in interpreting what is happening in the environment and in the body has been further clarified by some ingenious experiments by a psychologist called Schachter. In these experiments volunteers were given injections of either adrenalin or an inactive substance. Some of the subjects who had received adrenalin were correctly informed of the physiological reactions they should expect (such as tremor) while others were either incorrectly informed (that they would experience, for example, itching) or told nothing at all. Immediately after the injection each subject was placed in a waiting room, in which there was one of Schachter's accomplices. The accomplice proceeded to try to induce an emotional state in the subject, either anger, by being critical and irritable, or humour, by telling jokes and being light-hearted. Meanwhile the subject was observed through a one-way mirror.

Those subjects who had been misinformed or told nothing about the effect of the adrenalin injection showed a much greater emotional response than those who had been correctly informed or given the inert injection. They apparently attributed their physiological arousal to the behaviour of the accomplice, and therefore experienced the corresponding emotion. The correctly informed subjects attributed the same sensations to the impersonal, chemical effect of the injection, and experienced very little emotion. This and many other similar studies show that emotional states such as joy, anxiety and despair depend, not just on external events, but on our interpretation of our own physical sensations — which may have entirely different origins. We experience stress when our appraisal leads us to believe that the situation is threatening to our well-being. When our appraisal is correct the stress reaction is appropriate. When it is not we suffer quite needlessly.

Above: *This image of two men at the mercy of children armed with machine-guns is profoundly shocking. But what if you are told that it is a scene from a film, played by actors? In the same way, emotional responses to everyday stresses can be completely transformed by different preconceptions.*

no sound-track at all showed intermediate physiological arousal whilst the other two groups, who heard the neutral and positive commentaries, showed slightly

Our physical and bodily reactions to stress are mainly governed by our nervous system. This is a complex organization, and to understand stress reactions it is helpful to know its major divisions.

Broadly speaking, the nervous system has three divisions: those nerves which bring information from various parts of the body to the brain; the brain itself, which analyzes and organizes the information and decides on the response; and output nerves which take messages from the brain to different parts of the body.

Nerves are not the only route by which the brain receives or sends signals; certain centres in the brain and body organs are sensitive to 'chemical messengers' carried in the bloodstream called hormones. Glands in the brain secrete hormones directly into the blood when required, and these stimulate

Right: *Stress reactions such as sweating and gooseflesh are controlled by the sympathetic branch of the autonomic nervous system. The parasympathetic branch regulates the normal functions of the body in a relaxed state. Both the autonomic nervous system and the voluntary nervous system are controlled by the hypothalamus and the pituitary.*

the organs into acting appropriately.

The body has more than one output nervous system. One set of nerves controls our voluntary movements: these are the nerves which activate the muscles in the arm and hand when we raise a cup to the mouth. This is naturally called the voluntary nervous system. There is, however, a second nervous system, whose job it is to look after many body processes which are outside our

PHYSICAL SIGNS OF STRESS		
When confronted by a difficult, important or stressful situation do you:		
Get palpitations (racing heart)?	YES	NO
Get sweaty palms?	YES	NO
Get breathless?	YES	NO
Get headaches which feel like a tight band around your head?	YES	NO
Get diarrhoea?	YES	NO
Tremble in the legs, arms or hands?	YES	NO
Get 'butterflies in the stomach'?	YES	NO
Get a dry mouth?	YES	NO
Get a stiff or aching neck?	YES	NO
Clench your fists or your jaw?	YES	NO
All these are physical symptoms of stress, and if you answered 'yes' to a lot of the questions, then it is possible that your basic stress level is too high.		

PHYSICAL REACTIONS TO STRESS

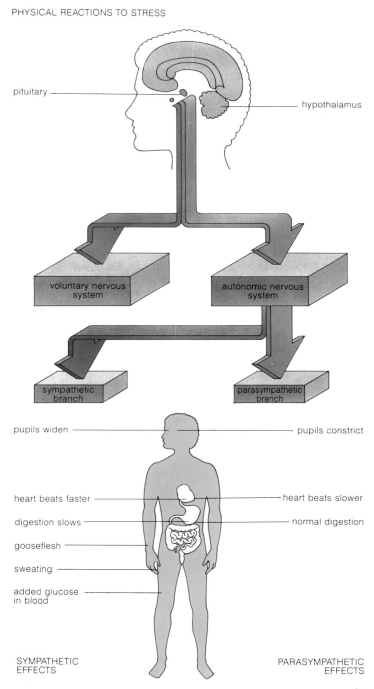

SYMPATHETIC
EFFECTS

PARASYMPATHETIC
EFFECTS

direct conscious control. This is the autonomic nervous system. There are many vital functions, such as heartbeat, breathing, digestion and temperature regulation, which are wholly or partly controlled by the nerves of the autonomic nervous system. In general terms, it is responsible for ensuring that the internal body processes maintain the correct level of activity, by making adjustments when necessary.

The autonomic nervous system itself is divided into two major branches—the sympathetic and parasympathetic branches. Most, but not all, internal organs have nerve connections to both of these branches.

The action of the sympathetic branch serves to prepare the whole body for an emergency. It provokes changes in the body mechanisms which make it ready for immediate energetic action: either to escape

BATTLE FATIGUE

Some of the most stressful conditions that a human being can encounter occur during battle. During World War I the numerous stress-related psychiatric casualties were thought to be suffering from the effect of explosion shock waves on the brain, and the condition was known as 'shell shock'. Views changed, though, and by the time of World War II the symptoms were recognized for what they were, and called war neurosis, battle fatigue, or combat exhaustion. The long-term effects suffered by veterans include depression, guilt, sleep disorders, alcoholism, drug-taking and even suicide.

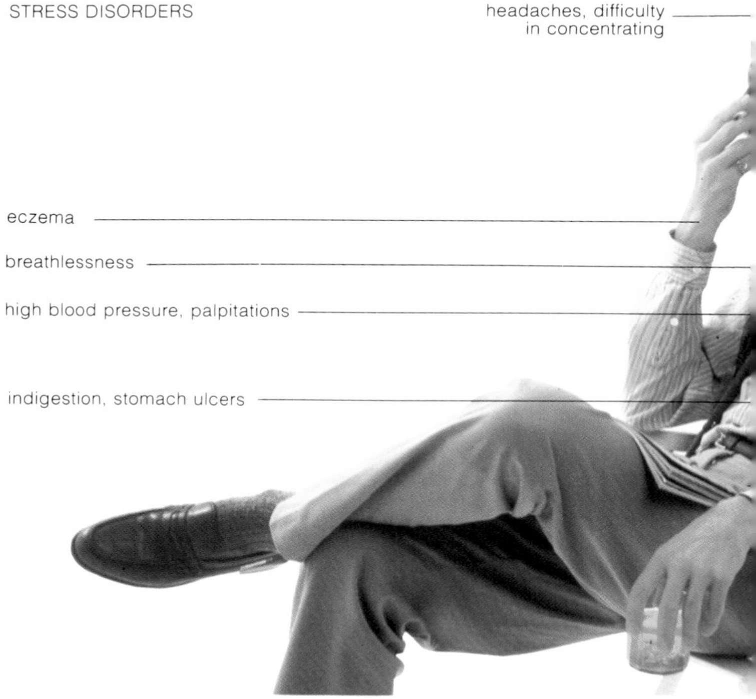

STRESS DISORDERS

headaches, difficulty _____
in concentrating

eczema ————————————————————

breathlessness ————————————————

high blood pressure, palpitations —————————————

indigestion, stomach ulcers ——————————

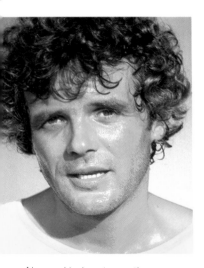

Above: *Under stress, the nervous system triggers reactions which are not consciously controllable.* Below: *Some of the many disorders caused by prolonged stress.*

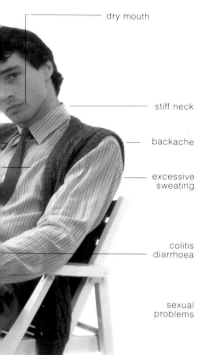

dry mouth

stiff neck

backache

excessive sweating

colitis
diarrhoea

sexual problems

from the threat or confront it. These two main options have been termed 'flight or fight'. When the sympathetic system is strongly activated the heart beats faster and stronger, the pupils of the eyes widen, digestion slows or stops, and more blood is pumped to the voluntary muscles and brain and less to the skin and gut. The skin perspires, and stored sugar products (giving energy) are delivered from the liver into the blood. All of these changes can be seen as giving a priority to immediate action, while processes which can wait, like digestion, are suspended.

The action of the parasympathetic branch is in many ways the opposite of the sympathetic. In fact it is through the opposition of the two branches that the internal balance (also called 'homeostasis') of the body is maintained. Under parasympathetic stimulation the heart slows, the pupils of the eyes constrict, the sweating response diminishes but salivation increases, the level of sugar products in the blood falls, and blood is directed away from the voluntary muscles toward the gut, which gets on with the job of digestion. In general, stress and anxiety are characterized by a preponderance of the sympathetic over the parasympathetic activity, whereas the opposite occurs during relaxation, rest and sleep.

The balance between the two branches of the autonomic nervous system is controlled by a group of interconnected nerve structures in the brain, which have been shown to be critical in determining emotional states. One of these structures, the hypothalamus, is particularly important. Studies have shown that electrical stimulation of certain parts of the hypothalamus activates the sympathetic system, whilst stimulation of other parts activates the parasympathetic system. In addition to secreting hormones, the hypothalamus also controls the action of the pituitary gland. (see page 37).

Psychologists and others have distinguished three broad patterns of behaviour among humans and animals in stressful situations. These are 'freezing', escape behaviour and aggression.

Freezing

Certain animals and birds, such as hares, rabbits and pheasants, will freeze when confronted with a sudden, unexpected danger. This has been described by one distinguished psychologist as 'silent, tense immobility'. It involves total immobility, silence, bristling of the hair, fur or feathers and defaecation. It is a highly active response, in that the musculature is very tense and the animal is totally alert. This is true even when the animal 'plays dead' — which may be thought of as an extreme form of freezing.

It has been suggested that the response serves certain animals well, enabling them to evade attacks from their predators through not drawing attention to themselves. The bristling of the fur may also make the animal look bigger and more dangerous to an attacker. Freezing as a stress response is common among certain animal species, but it is uncommon in humans. Even those animals which

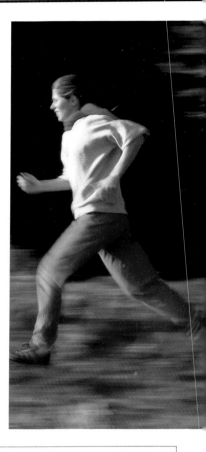

GIVING UP SMOKING

Increased smoking is a common symptom of stress. For the smoker, it is only too easy to reach for another cigarette to steady the nerves. The sedative effect of smoking is insignificant, though, compared to the damage it does. The risk of lung cancer among smokers is nine times that among non-smokers, and the risk of heart attack is doubled. For anyone who values his or her health, it is essential to give up.

There is no single way to give up smoking which can be recommended for everyone. Different methods suit different people. As a general rule, however, giving up suddenly is more effective than giving up gradually. Set a date, such as New Year's Eve, when you will stop smoking completely. Merely reducing the number of cigarettes you smoke or converting to low-tar brands is far less effective from the health point of view, and it is easy to slip back into old habits if you still smoke occasionally. Identify danger periods, such as after meals or at parties, when you particularly want to smoke, and develop alternative responses to the craving such as eating fruit or drinking water. Using chewing gum containing nicotine may help.

do freeze readily are unlikely to do so if escape is possible.

Escape

For certain animals, birds and fish, escape is a virtually automatic response to danger. In humans it is far from automatic, but when we judge that the threat is greater than our capacity to handle it, 'flight' is a natural and often successful reaction. Escape behaviour may take several forms; a holiday may be a form of escape from a taxing or boring job.

A closely related response is avoidance, which means not entering into a situation which we anticipate will contain a threat. For example, a child who anticipates that some aspect of school will be unpleasant may well try to avoid it by staying at home. Fear or panic are frequent accompaniments of escape behaviour, whilst anxiety is the typical hallmark of avoidance.

Left: *Escape is one of the most basic behavioural responses to stress, although most people need to be in a real panic before they actually start running.*
Below: *Consumption disorders such as compulsive eating and excessive drinking are common reactions to stress.*

Aggression

Normally placid animals when subjected to the stress of overcrowding will show various forms of aggressive behaviour, including biting, rearing and threatening displays. In humans, aggression is particularly associated with two circumstances. As was described on page 13, aggressiveness, hostility and irritability is a pattern of emotional reaction displayed by some patients immediately after they have undergone surgery. The other area in which stress-related aggressive behaviour may be seen is in certain personality types, characteristically hard-driving individuals who work at high pressure. This personality type has been called 'Type A' (see page 30) and it includes elements of aggressiveness and competitiveness.

Consumption disorders

Finally, another group of stress-related behaviours, some of which are seen only in humans, involves eating, swallowing or otherwise taking things into the body. Smoking, drinking, over-eating, under-eating and the taking of medicines or other drugs are all behavioural patterns which may be associated with stress.

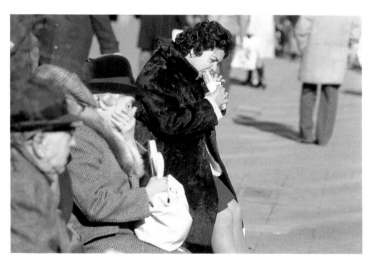

THE HEALTH RISK

In the following pages we shall look at some of the main ways in which stress is related to health and disease. Stress can be responsible for bringing an illness on, or it can cause a 'flare-up' or worsening of some existing condition. Broadly speaking, stress affects behaviour, physical functioning and emotional experience—usually all three together. If the stress is sufficient to affect health, the consequences can be similarly divided into these three areas.

Behaviour

The most important stress-related behaviours which affect health are those which involve consumption— that is, taking substances into the body. Stress can alter eating patterns and consequently weight. Some people over-eat as a response to stress, and may become overweight (obese). This leads to dissatisfaction with one's appearance, and puts a strain on the heart. Conversely, stress can also lead to severe loss of appetite and under-eating (anorexia).

Smoking is another stress-related form of behaviour: analysis of smoking patterns clearly shows the connection between periods of stress and 'lighting up'. Smoking is

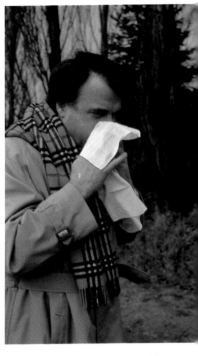

Above: *Under stress the body's natural immunity to infection is reduced, and people become more vulnerable to colds and 'flu.*

STOMACH ULCERS

Digestion is achieved by acid in the stomach breaking down food. Normally, the stomach secretes acid in appropriate amounts when it is needed, and then stops when the task of digestion is complete. The parasympathetic branch of the autonomic nervous system (see page 22) controls acid secretion. Under stress the acid is produced in great quantities and at times that it is not needed, with no food to work on, it erodes the lining of the stomach and produces an ulcer. Ulcers are more common in men than women, and it has been estimated that in industrialized countries, ten per cent of the population will suffer from stomach ulcers at some time in their lives.

The basic treatment for ulcers involves regulating the diet (reducing consumption of irritant or indigestible food), reducing alcohol intake, and adjusting eating habits (eating more slowly, for example, and not eating while working). It is recognized, however, that taking steps to combat stress can speed up the healing process, and also prevent ulcers forming. Comparison of stressed laboratory animals has shown that, while equally stressed, those animals which were able to make effective responses which altered their situation developed fewer ulcers.

not in itself an illness, but it is a major contributor to many serious diseases. The link between smoking and lung cancer is now common knowledge, but the fact that smoking is one of the main causes of premature death from heart disease is perhaps less well known.

Physical functioning
It has been shown that many physical illnesses are partially caused or made worse by stress. They include heart disease, digestive disorders such as stomach ulcers and ulcerative colitis, allergies such as asthma, and skin disorders such as eczema. Stress can also lower the body's resistance to infection, making the individual vulnerable to colds and influenza as well as more serious diseases. This comes about through changes in the immune system which is responsible for organising the body's response to the presence of foreign objects like bacteria, viruses, fungi and tumours, as well as tissue grafts and organ transplants. The cells which attack alien objects, called lymphocytes, are grown in the bone marrow and located in the blood and tissues. Stress interferes with the immune system by reducing the overall number of available lymphocytes. Experiments with artificially stressed animals have shown reduced lymphocyte levels, and an increased risk of illness and death. In humans, similar impairment of the immune system has been found in severely depressed patients and in the bereaved.

Emotional experiences
The emotional effects of stress, which most of us will be able to identify from our own personal experience, may be grouped under the two broad headings of anxiety (including fears and phobias) and depression. When these are severe they can cause sleep disorders and reduced work efficiency. Anxiety and depression are often accompanied by impaired alertness and concentration, which may in turn lead to mental lapses. In this way, stress has been held partly responsible for the occurrence of accidents in the home, at work, and on the road. Stress may be a contributory factor to 'accident proneness'.

Below: *Smokers get through a lot more cigarettes when they are anxious. Stress can, indirectly, be a major health hazard.*

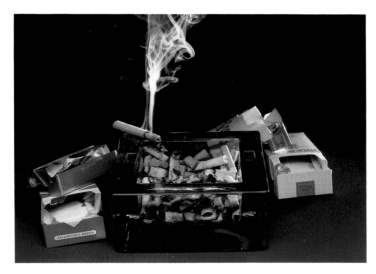

One of the main causes of premature deaths in developed countries of Western Europe, the USA and Australia is heart disease. Although this epidemic has been brought under partial control by people giving up smoking and eating more healthy foods, it is still a major problem, and stress has been identified as a contributory factor.

Heart attacks occur when the pumping muscle of the heart is starved of oxygen. This causes pain, damage, and can ultimately lead to death. It has been known for many years that smoking, lack of exercise, obesity and the eating of fatty foods increases the risk of heart attacks greatly. Stress also increases the risk.

Stress is associated with increased activity of the sympathetic nervous system (see page 22). One of the things that this does is to release free fatty acids

Below: *Under stress the sympathetic nervous system becomes more active and stimulates physical reactions such as faster heartbeat and slowed digestion. It also makes the liver produce more cholesterol which, deposited in the coronary arteries, can cause a heart attack.*

into the bloodstream. These free fatty acids can be converted into into cholesterol which is deposited on the inside surfaces of blood vessels, especially the large arteries supplying the heart muscle which are called the coronary arteries. It is the clogging up of these arteries which causes the oxygen starvation of the heart muscle.

The clogging process is speeded up when the pressure of the blood within the blood vessels is high. Blood pressure goes up and down depending upon what we are doing: when we are physically active it goes up and when we rest or sleep it goes down. If the pressure is permanently high it puts a strain on the arteries and makes them more vulnerable to damage. This makes them more likely to become coated and clogged. The condition when the blood pressure is raised all or most of the time is also known as hypertension. It leads to a vicious cycle in which the heart must pump harder to force the blood around the body. This in turn leads to the heart muscle increasing in size, which increases its need for oxygen. Because the clogged arteries cannot deliver blood in sufficient quantities to keep pace with the heart's need for oxygen, the

STRESS AND CORONARY ARTERY DISEASE

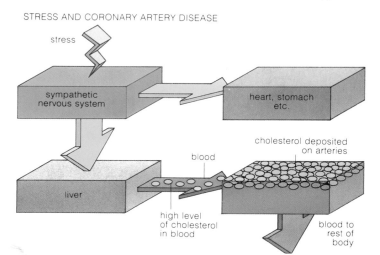

stress

sympathetic nervous system

heart, stomach etc.

cholesterol deposited on arteries

blood

liver

high level of cholesterol in blood

blood to rest of body

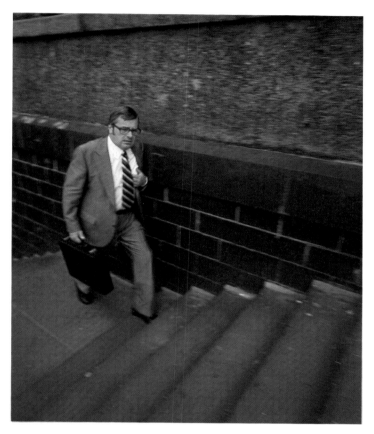

Above: *Heart disease is a major killer in the West, and it is believed that high stress levels significantly increase the risk of attack.*

chances of a heart attack are greatly increased.

Hypertension can lead to problems elsewhere in the body too. The kidneys, which help to control and adjust blood pressure, can become damaged. The high blood pressure can also force one of the weakened blood vessels to 'spring a leak'. When this happens in the brain it is known as a stroke.

One of the earliest studies into the effect of stress on coronary heart disease showed that prolonged stress, especially when associated with a high degree of work responsibility, affected over 90 per cent of a group of coronary patients. This compared with only 20 per cent in a healthy group of similar age, race and occupation. Overwork, such as having two jobs, or working very long hours, also appeared to increase the risk of heart attacks. It is small wonder, then, that company directors have exceptionally high rates of coronary heart disease, while those whose jobs involve more reasonable working hours, such as gardeners and clergymen, are among the lowest risk groups for this condition. Accountants are more likely to have their attacks when the end of the financial year is approaching, when they are under considerable stress.

While it has been demonstrated that smoking, diet, age, and exercise are the principal factors which make heart attacks more likely, many doctors have observed that a particular type of personality or temperament is common among coronary victims.

Research conducted by two heart specialists, Dr Meyer Friedman and Dr Ray Rosenman, has led to a clear description of the coronary-prone personality, which they termed the 'Type A' personality. The characteristics of the Type A individual are:
• A strong and prolonged drive to achieve personal goals which are poorly defined.
• A strong desire to compete.
• A strong desire for self-improvement, success and recognition.
• A tendency to attempt too many different things in too little time.
• A tendency to do things as quickly as possible.
• A high level of mental and physical alertness.

It is apparent from this that the Type A individual is ambitious and motivated to compete and achieve. He or she tends to do things quickly and to operate under time pressure. Generally this person is always highly aroused and 'on the go'.

The questionnaire which appears on the opposite page will allow you to judge how similar you are to the personality type that Friedman and Rosenman described.

If you have a Type A personality, it is possible to modify your behaviour and perhaps reduce the risk of heart trouble. The various approaches described do not attempt to resolve underlying problems and worries, but concentrate on reviewing priorities, self-observation, alternative ways of responding to stress, and relaxation.

Reviewing priorities

Try to establish long-term goals both in your work and in your private life. See if you can set aside some time for solitude and contemplation, instead of always being busy and rushing about. Ask yourself if all the things that you are doing have to be done right now.

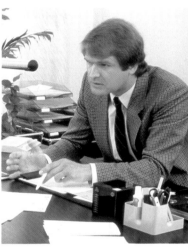

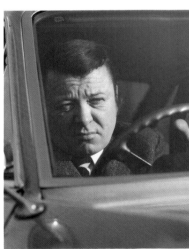

Above right: *Ambitious, impatient, competitive 'Type A' personalities tend to be more vulnerable to heart attacks than less highly-pressured people.*
Right: *Frustrating situations like traffic jams can increase the risk; it is important to learn how to simmer down and relax.*

Self-observation

You must become aware of which kinds of situations 'wind you up'. Typical examples are being stuck in a traffic jam, waiting in a slow-moving queue and being interrupted in whatever you are doing by the telephone ringing.

Alternative ways of responding

Instead of responding to problems with frustration and aggressiveness you should learn to do two things. First, you should consider whether the situation is really so important. Do you really need to take it so seriously and get so worked up? Second, you can practise responding differently. For example, if you find yourself in a traffic jam you can respond by turning on the car radio to listen to relaxing music.

Relaxation

Regular practise of relaxation techniques such as those described on pages 60-61 will also be helpful.

DO YOU HAVE A TYPE A PERSONALITY?		
Do you do most things as quickly as you can?	YES	NO
Do you have a short temper?	YES	NO
Do you take work home at weekends or on holiday?	YES	NO
Do you try to do more than one thing at a time?	YES	NO
Do you find it hard to tolerate delays, as in queues or traffic jams?	YES	NO
Do you prefer competitive games and sports to non-competitive ones?	YES	NO
Are you impatient when you see someone doing something slower than you could do it?	YES	NO
Do you smoke?	YES	NO
Do you always rise to a challenge?	YES	NO
Are you fascinated by numbers and amounts, and do you like to accumulate things?	YES	NO
Do you feel a little guilty when you relax or do nothing?	YES	NO
Do you believe that if you want a job done well you must do it yourself?	YES	NO
The more questions you answered 'yes', the more you have a Type A personality. Your health might be at risk, and you are probably not getting as much out of life as you could. You should consider making some adjustments to your behaviour patterns.		

ALCOHOL

Alcohol, consumed in moderation, is a universal, socially-accepted drink which helps people unwind and promotes easy social interaction. It acts as a 'cerebral depressant', which means that it suppresses the activity of that part of the brain called the cerebral cortex, allowing drives and impulses more freedom of expression. After a few drinks, people feel less shy and inhibited, less worried generally, more confident and more able to enjoy themselves. Occasional drinking of moderate amounts of alcohol is a harmless part of normal social behaviour.

The use of alcohol becomes a problem when a person comes to rely upon it for certain effects. These effects may include the emotional lift which gives relief from boredom and depression; freedom from stress or tension; even oblivion and sleep. It is important to understand that alcohol is a drug, like those described on the previous pages, and as with all drugs it has its negative effects and disadvantages. Unfortunately, owing to the easy availability of alcohol and its well-known positive effects, alcohol-related problems are very common indeed.

Alcohol can produce true physiological addiction, which has a number of characteristic symptoms: Alcohol comes to dominate the individual's life. A period of abstinence will provoke a withdrawal state which involves tremor ('the shakes'), sweating and nausea. 'Tolerance' develops,

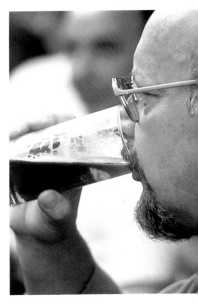

Above: *For most people, alcohol is a harmless social pleasure, which helps them relax and unwind. For those who rely on it, though, it is a dangerous drug.*

meaning that larger amounts of alcohol can be consumed without the obvious signs of intoxication appearing. There will also be a compulsion to drink, which may be experienced as craving or loss of control. Addiction and dependence are not necessarily the same thing. Many people who misuse alcohol and rely on it may not be fully addicted in the sense described. Either way, the social and

---

WHAT IS A SAFE LEVEL OF DRINKING?

Medical research has shown that drinking will seriously damage your health if you consume more than about four pints (2.3 litres) of beer, or four double measures of spirits, or one 70cl bottle of wine per day. Such levels are well above the sensible maximum, however, and if you regularly drink at this rate, you have a problem. In practice, one pint (0.57 litres) of beer, one double measure of spirits, or a glass and a half of wine are reasonable limits for men. Women have a lower threshold, and should reduce these limits by a third. These are average figures: if you drink more on some days, drink less on others.

ALCOHOL-RELATED MORTALITY

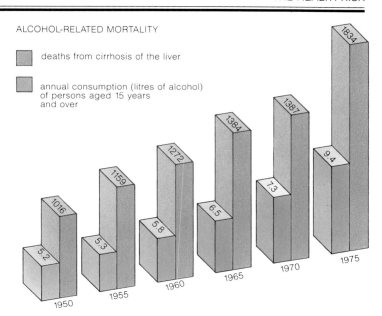

deaths from cirrhosis of the liver

annual consumption (litres of alcohol)
of persons aged 15 years
and over

Above: *The steady rise in alcohol consumption since 1950 is mirrored by the death rate from cirrhosis of the liver—just one of the risks run by heavy drinkers.*

personal costs of alcohol misuse are high. The positive, mood-raising effects are only present at low doses of up to about 50 milligrams in 100 millilitres (50mg/100ml) in the blood. This level can be reached by drinking as little as 1½ pints of beer. At higher blood alcohol levels (around 100mg/100ml) slurred speech and clumsiness appear, and at higher levels, stupor, coma and eventually death.

Alcohol is certainly responsible for a great deal of death and injury on the roads. Even at the British legal limit of 80mg/100ml it has been estimated that the risk of a road accident is twice the risk run by sober drivers.

In broad terms, alcohol can lead to three main kinds of problems for the drinker: social problems, mental problems and physical problems. The social problems include broken marriage, sexual difficulties, loss of friends,

unemployment and trouble with the law. Mental disabilities may be of two kinds. Emotional problems such as gloom and self-doubt can develop after prolonged heavy drinking. More seriously, the chemical effects of alcohol on the brain may lead to brain damage involving impaired thinking and poor memory. The physical problems mainly concern the liver and the digestive system, as well as the brain, all of which become damaged through prolonged high alcohol consumption. In addition, an unborn child will be adversely affected by high alcohol levels in its mother's bloodstream.

The many severe dangers associated with alcohol make it a risky choice as a stress-relieving agent. Indeed, problem drinking can be as stressful as the problems which provoked the drinking in the first place.

Fortunately there are sources of help for people with drinking problems. Help may come from the 'official' health carers, such as family doctors and psychiatrists, or from self-help organisations such as Alcoholics Anonymous.

The main defining element of depression is a feeling of great sadness, but a depressive state will usually involve much more besides. The depressed person may have a poor opinion of himself or herself, even to the extent of feeling worthless. The future may appear bleak and unpromising, and the world may take on a joyless or meaningless aspect. The depressed individual may be tearful, lethargic, tired, withdrawn, sleepless, irritable and tense. He or she may have thoughts of suicide.

Family doctors, psychiatrists and hospital services are very familiar with the depressed patient, but a fact that has only recently come to light is that there are many people in society who, although not in contact with medical or social services, are equally depressed. One survey of women in a deprived inner suburb of a large city found that 15 per cent of them were suffering from depression, and an additional 18 per cent were borderline cases.

This study, conducted by two sociologists, George Brown and Tirril Harris, was able to go a long way in showing the role of past and current stresses in the emergence of depression in women. Through careful interviewing they were able to identify a number of contributory factors in the depressed womens' circumstances and backgrounds.

Brown and Harris found three groups of factors associated with depression in women. One group, the provoking factors, determined *when* a depressive episode began. A second group, the vulnerability factors, determined *who* developed depression. A third group, the severity factors, explained the type or severity of the condition.

Provoking factors
Provoking factors were of two kinds. Life events, such as those described on page 14, were important, although only certain types seemed to contribute to depression. Severe life events, which lasted for a considerable

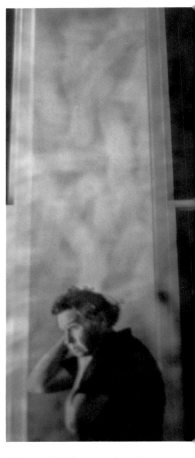

Above: *A high proportion of depressives suffer alone, too withdrawn or lethargic to seek professional help.*

period of time (a week or longer) and which involved some sort of actual or threatened loss, were most often associated with depressive states. The second group of provoking or formative factors were so-called major difficulties. These consisted of persistent adverse circumstances, such as housing or financial problems.

Vulnerability factors
The factors that identified which

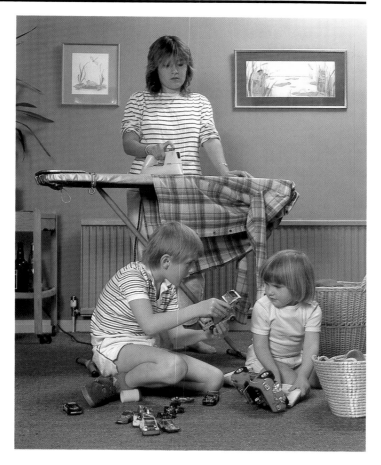

Above: *The constant strain of looking after several small children makes mothers particularly vulnerable to depression.*

women would be susceptible to the impact of severe life events or major difficulties were: lack of a close and confiding relationship with a husband or boyfriend; the loss of the mother, but not of the father, through death or other cause before the age of eleven; and the presence of three or more children aged 14 or less in the home.

Severity factors

Depressions were more severe if an additional severe life event occurred after the depressive episode had begun; or if the woman had had a previous loss of either parent, brother or sister, child or husband, in childhood, adolescence or adulthood. There was evidence that depressive states in those who had experienced loss by death were more severe than in those who had experienced loss by separation. Even though the results of this research relate only to women living in a deprived inner city area, it probably has wider significance. The research demonstrates the link between emotional disorder and a variety of life stresses both present and past, short term and long term.

35

It has been recognized for a long time by doctors and others that prolonged stress can have adverse effects on general health. One of the earliest scientific theories to explain this relationship was proposed by Dr Hans Selye in the late 1940s. He observed that experimentally stressed rats developed characteristic health problems, such as stomach ulcers. Patients with a variety of physical diseases also showed a characteristic reaction to the stress of illness, including loss of appetite and vitality. He suggested that there was a standard sequence of stages which animals and people go through irrespective of the source of the stress. His model of the stress response is known as the General Adaptation Syndrome, which emphasizes the idea that it concerns the organism's way of adapting to stress over a long period.

Seyle proposed that there are three stages which a person goes through when exposed to stress for a prolonged period of time. Stage one is called the 'alarm reaction': a short-lived stage during which the person's psychological and physical resources are mobilised to deal with the immediate emergency. If the stress persists, this is followed by stage two, known as the 'resistance' stage. During this stage the individual's physical resistance to stress is in fact superior to the normal resting level. This means that the body's internal defences are mobilized and maintained at a higher level than usual. Stage three is 'exhaustion' and is the final stage when stress is very prolonged. The body's energy supplies, which have been used to keep its physical defences geared up to a high pitch, are exhausted; the result is collapse, vulnerability to infection and disease, or even, in extreme cases, death.

In addition to describing these three stages; Selye suggested what the physical process underlying

Below: *Resistance to stress alters dramatically if the stress-producing conditions persist for a long time. The response curve of the General Adaptation Syndrome shows how, during the initial alarm phase, stress resistance drops below normal, but then rises, enabling the stressor to be dealt with. Eventually, though, exhaustion saps the body's ability to resist.*

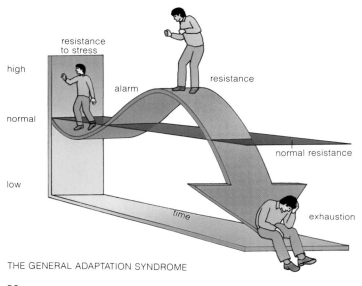

high

normal

low

resistance to stress

alarm

resistance

normal resistance

time

exhaustion

THE GENERAL ADAPTATION SYNDROME

THE EFFECTS OF PROLONGED STRESS

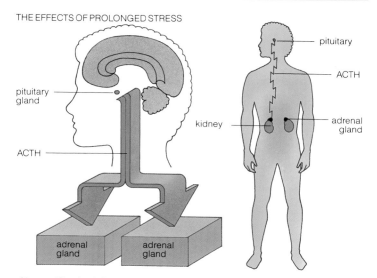

Above: *The body's reactions to stress are stimulated by the adrenal system. The process is triggered by the pituitary gland, which responds to stress signals by releasing the hormone ACTH into the blood. This is carried to the adrenal glands, and these react by producing the adrenalin which, carried in the blood, energizes the body for instant action.*

Constant noise is a powerful source of prolonged stress, and a survey of people living near Los Angeles International Airport found that they had higher rates of blood pressure, heart disease and even suicide compared to similar people living in quieter areas.

them might be. The process he proposed is a complicated one, mainly concerned with the levels of hormones circulating in the blood and with the glands which produce these hormones. (A hormone is a substance which is produced in one part of the body and has its effect in another part. Hormones have been called 'chemical messengers'.)

The brain, which registers the stressful event or situation, immediately stimulates the pituitary gland which is a small structure located deep within the brain itself. One of the substances released into the blood by the pituitary gland is the adrenocorticotrophic hormone, usually shortened to ACTH. The ACTH travels round the bloodstream and reaches the adrenal glands which are sited on

the top part of both kidneys. The ACTH stimulates the adrenal glands to release adrenalin into the blood, and this has a number of energizing effects, including raising heart rate, blood pressure, and improving muscle tone.

Selye also noticed that post-mortems of animals which had been exposed to prolonged stress revealed that the adrenal glands had changed in colour and size, being shrunken and darkened. This suggested to him that they had been overworked and 'burned out'. This overworking of the pituitary—adrenal chemical system has been regarded as a factor in the development of certain psychosomatic or 'stress' diseases such as coronary heart disease, stomach ulcers and some skin disorders such as eczema.

Fears and phobias have to do with the perception of danger. Everyone will have experienced fear and will know that it is the unpleasant feeling we get when we come up against something that will do us harm. Obviously, the ability to experience fear is a very useful reaction to us; it alerts us to the need to take some kind of immediate action—either to run away ('flight') or to confront the danger and eliminate it ('fight').

Phobias are exaggerated and unreasonable fears. If someone reacts to something as if it were dangerous, when in reality it isn't, we speak of a phobia. In all of the common phobias the degree of fear the individual experiences is quite out of proportion to the actual danger. Another way in which phobias are different from fears lies in the severity of the reaction itself. Ordinary fears are associated with moderate degrees of fearfulness, dislike and aversion, but with phobias the level of emotional disturbance can be crippling in its severity. People with phobias sometimes reach a state of panic, whereas those with simple fears rarely do.

The final ingredient of a phobia is avoidance. It is part of ordinary commonsense to keep away from dangers, but the phobic individual

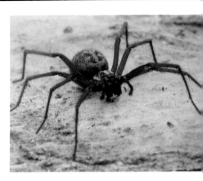

Above: *A harmless spider can produce total panic in some people—a very common example of specific phobia.*
Right: *Everyday activities such as visiting the local shopping centre can become a nightmare to the agoraphobic. Such fears can disrupt one's whole way of life.*

is acutely conscious of the possibility of coming into contact with whatever it is that they cannot tolerate. For example, a person with a spider phobia may avoid going into the bathroom in case there is a spider in the bath.

Types of phobia
There are three main groups of phobias: specific phobias, social

---

SELF-HELP FOR FIGHTING PHOBIAS

If you suffer from a phobia you can do a lot to help yourself. Just what you should do depends upon the type of phobia you have, but the common element in all forms of help is exposure to, or confrontation with whatever it is that is feared. This obviously takes a lot of self-discipline, and it is important to do it gradually. In the case of specific phobias such as fear of certain animals, gradual confrontation may be achieved using pictures before moving on to the real thing. The gradual approach may also be used to combat social phobias, by practising handling simulated social situations with sympathetic friends before trying 'real life' situations.

If you are agoraphobic, try longer and longer trips from home or journeys on public transport, first accompanied and later unaccompanied. Keeping a diary of your achievements will help you to monitor progress. Understanding the mental and physical mechanisms of anxiety and fear will help to make these feelings tolerable. All of the above approaches may be combined with relaxation techniques and cognitive methods (see pages 60 and 70).

phobias and agoraphobia. Specific phobias involve distinct objects, animals or defined situations. Some of the commonest specific phobias are of spiders, snakes, insects, birds, dentists, injections, flying, thunderstorms, heights and enclosed spaces. Examples of social phobias are parties, public speaking, eating in public places and interacting in any way with the opposite sex.

The third main group of phobic disorders is agoraphobia. This term derives from the Greek word *agora* meaning a market place. Agoraphobia is sometimes thought to mean a fear of wide open spaces, but in fact it is a much more complicated and troublesome condition than its name implies. Agoraphobia is really a set of problems centering around a fear of being away from home by oneself. This fear is often associated with a fear of enclosed places (claustrophobia) and a fear of travelling by public transport. For

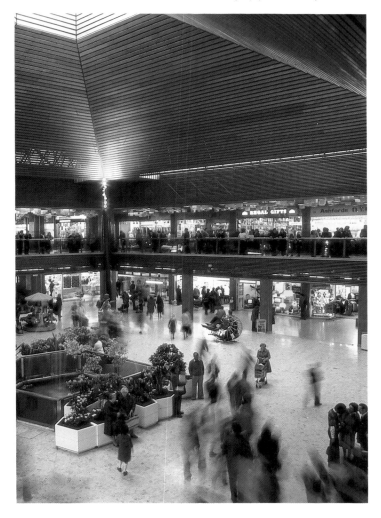

many agoraphobics their greatest fear is of being overcome by extreme anxiety or panic whilst away from home and being unable to get back. Agoraphobics will often have other phobias, particularly social phobias, as well. In addition, the social isolation that agoraphobia leads to can result in loneliness and depression.

What causes phobias?

For a long time it was widely believed that phobias developed from *learned* reactions. Countless experiments with animals showed that if they were repeatedly frightened or shocked in conjunction with some neutral stimulus, then after a while they developed a phobic avoidance reaction to the stimulus which had previously been neutral for them. For example, repeated mild electric shocks preceded by the sounding of a buzzer led to a state where the sounding of the buzzer alone was enough to get the animal showing stress and attempting to escape from the situation. It was assumed that human phobias had been acquired in a similar way.

This 'learning' theory was very helpful to psychologists, because it led directly to forms of treatment (see page 41) which proved most effective. Recent work, however, indicates that the learning theory is unable to explain satisfactorily certain aspects of human phobias.

Firstly, unlike animals, people are quite resistant to experimentally induced fears. Secondly, the vast majority of people who have undergone extremely frightening, traumatic experiences do not develop lasting fears, while the learning approach predicts that they ought to. Thirdly, the 'learned reaction' theory would predict that *any* neutral object could be turned into a phobic object, given the right conditions, but this is not the case. Some things which are associated with real dangers in their own right, such as cars, almost never become the focus of phobias; others, such as spiders, which we see many

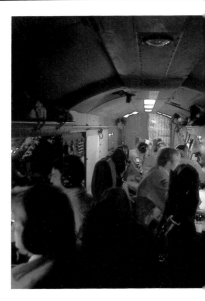

Above: *Complete freedom from claustrophobia—fear of enclosed spaces—is a basic qualification for working on a submarine.*

fewer of and are generally harmless, frequently become the subject of phobias. Furthermore, most people with phobias have not gone through repeated traumatic experiences like the animals described above.

Direct learning probably plays a part in the origin of some phobias, but other processes are at work as well. We get many of our emotional responses through observing others. For example, there is a tendency for children whose mothers have a phobia to develop the same phobia themselves. We also develop fear reactions when we obtain information that something is dangerous. It is not difficult to imagine that being told by a usually reliable individual that something (a dog) or a class of things (all dogs) will bite you could easily lead to fearfulness.

Fear reduction

Obviously, the treatment of a phobia will vary according to the nature of the fear itself—one would not go about overcoming a fear of snakes in the same way as a fear of public speaking. Nevertheless there are a number of methods that are applicable to different kinds of fears, which can be used singly or in combination to reduce or even eliminate a variety of phobias.

Systematic desensitization
This technique involves teaching the phobic person how to relax (see page 60) and then exposing him or her to a graded series of feared scenes or objects, starting with the easiest ones. In the case of a spider phobia the series might start with pictures of spiders, progressing through small dead spiders and ending up with larger live ones. The powerful effect of relaxation will act to neutralise the fear associated with each item in the series. This has proved to be a highly successful

method for treating a wide variety of specific phobias.

Flooding
In contrast to the gradual approach of systematic desensitization, flooding involves prolonged exposure to the feared object. This can be done either with 'real life' situations or with imagined ones, in which case the technique is known as implosion. These methods work because experience has shown that even very intense fears naturally subside after prolonged exposure of several hours duration.

Modelling
This involves observing a non-fearful person in contact with the feared object, and then imitating that person. This is the process by which most children lose their childhood fears. The fearful person has the opportunity to learn more appropriate ways of behaving toward and dealing with the feared object; in addition, unhelpful responses can be suppressed.

Below: *Many things in life depend on social contacts. People with social phobias miss out, and can easily lapse into depression.*

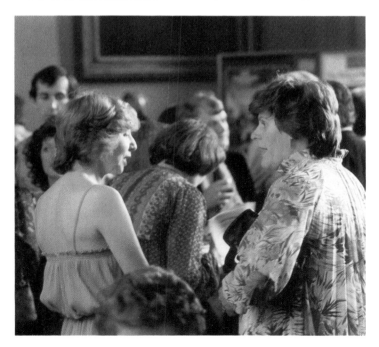

OCCUPATIONAL STRESS ━━━

Stress seems to be an inescapable part of going to work. This is not simply because work involves unacceptable pressures — it is also because stress of some sort is essential to efficiency. Such stress can be compared to the force applied to a simple tool like a tyre lever. If there is too little force, nothing will be achieved. If there is too much, something may be damaged. If the right amount of force is applied, however, the job is done quickly and efficiently. The effect of different levels of stress on human performance is very similar.

To understand the relationship between stress and performance it is helpful to measure the way stress activates certain bodily systems. This effect is called arousal, and it can be measured by a variety of techniques, such as detecting increases in perspiration rate or heart rate. Experiments involving such measurements have demonstrated that each of us functions at our best when we experience a moderate degree of arousal, which is in turn induced by

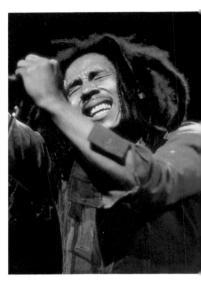

Above: *Inspired performers often achieve very high arousal levels, which may lead to exhaustion.*
Below: *In contrast an orchestral conductor must avoid over-arousal if he is to remain in control.*

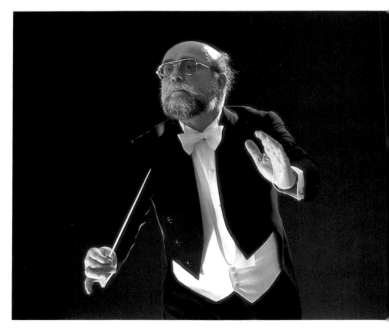

STRESS AND EFFICIENCY

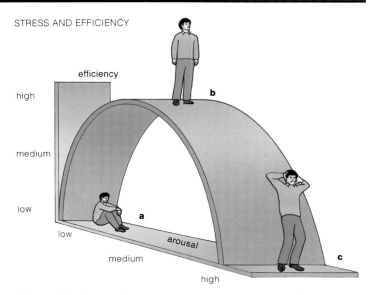

Above: *Efficiency suffers at low levels of arousal* (a) *but rises to a peak at moderate levels* (b). *Beyond this point further arousal results in confusion, and efficiency falls off again* (c).

a moderate degree of stress.

If arousal is too low we are not alert enough to perform well. When we are over-aroused we may notice certain exaggerated bodily reactions, such as a fast heart rate or rapid breathing. It becomes increasingly difficult to filter out irrelevant messages from our senses, so generally we find it difficult to concentrate. Our ability to perform efficiently, especially if the task is difficult, complicated or unfamiliar, is badly affected. Even well-rehearsed procedures may break down under conditions of high arousal. For example, under the extreme stress of battle a high percentage of soldiers are unable to carry out the practised sequence of loading and firing their weapons. Their efficiency is greatly reduced by heightened arousal which causes them to be either frozen with fear or disorganized and agitated.

As you might expect, easy tasks are much less prone to disruption by such high levels of arousal than difficult tasks. Thus, in a panic, a person would probably still be able to give his telephone number, but might well be incapable of solving a mental arithmetic problem, which is much more difficult. You do not have to be fighting in a battle zone to suffer in this way. A number of common factors have been discovered which can cause prolonged high levels of arousal. These include excessive time pressures, loss of sleep, inescapable demands imposed by other people, and a high incidence of life events (see page 14).

Normally, a person's level of arousal varies a great deal, from sleeping to waking, from relaxing to working. Unexpected and unfamiliar occurrences will tend to push the level of arousal up, which initially improves performance and makes problem-solving easier. A person who feels he or she is under stress, however, is usually aroused to the point of exhaustion, and is therefore not being as efficient as he or she could be. There are a number of things such a person might do to combat this, such as taking certain medications or practising relaxation techniques.

Most of us experience interviews, examinations or tests as fairly stressful. In some people the anxiety can be so intense that their performance during the test itself does not do them justice, and they may fail even though their real ability was good enough for them to have passed. High stress levels may also lead the examinee to fall ill or withdraw for other reasons before the exam. In a competitive society, with considerable rewards for success and ambition, the pressures on students can be very great. Ruined careers, and even suicides, have been blamed on test anxiety.

Simple tests consisting of short lists of questions are available to measure and gain a greater understanding of test anxiety. In one such study, two groups of university students, one group high in measured test anxiety and the other low, were each divided into five levels of ability. Only very small differences in exam results were found between the confident and the anxious students at the highest and lowest ability levels. In other words, the most able students tended to do well irrespective of test anxiety, while the students of low ability all performed equally poorly. In the intermediate ranges of ability, however, high test anxiety was associated with significantly poorer exam results. Not only did the more anxious students do worse in their exams, but about 20 per cent failed to complete their whole course of study, compared to about six per cent of the more confident students.

TEST ANXIETY				
	Almost never	Some-times	Often	Almost always
I get an uneasy, upset feeling when taking exams	1	2	3	4
During tests, I feel very tense	1	2	3	4
I feel panicky when I take an important test	1	2	3	4
I feel my heart beating fast during an important test	1	2	3	4
Thinking about the mark I may get in a course interferes with my work on tests	1	2	3	4
During exams I find myself thinking about whether I'll ever get through the course	1	2	3	4
Thoughts of failing interfere with my concentration on tests	1	2	3	4
During tests I find myself thinking about what will happen if I fail	1	2	3	4

Add up your scores on the first four questions (emotionality) and the last four (worry). If you have scored more than 10 on either the emotionality or worry sections then it is possible that test anxiety is affecting your performance during tests.

The stresses associated with exams, tests and interviews are similar to the extent that, in all of these situations, the individual feels that he or she is being evaluated or judged. Often, the poor test performance of an anxious examinee is associated with a personal sense of threat generated by the fear of failure. The same tasks can usually be performed much better by such people when the situation is not regarded as an evaluation or test.

It is now widely thought that test anxiety is made up of two components. On the one hand there are the physical reactions, as described on pages 20-23. On the other hand there are the mental reactions, which are usually self-critical and pessimistic.

Below: *For the anxious applicant, an interview with a prospective employer can seem like a judgement on his or her whole career and personality. The sense of threat can make quite capable people appear inadequate.*

The evidence suggests that it is the mental reactions which do most of the damage to the test performance of the person who suffers a high degree of text anxiety. Such students spend much of the test time worrying about their performance and the likelihood that others are doing better than they are. It is the distracting effect of worry, self-critical thoughts and anticipation of failure which interfere with concentration, making it difficult to think clearly and produce one's best work.

People with troublesome levels of test anxiety can often be helped. The kind of approach will depend upon whether the test anxiety is part of a more widespread group of anxiety problems, or whether it is a relatively isolated problem. If it is relatively isolated, a desensitization approach (see page 41) can prove helpful. If it is part of a more widespread condition, a broader and perhaps deeper method will be required, in which the person's various fears and worries may need to be explored.

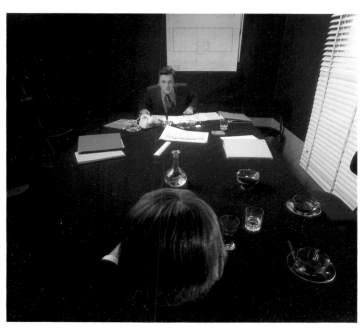

For many of us our jobs are an important source of stress. Surveys have shown that tens of millions of man-days per year are lost through nervous or emotional problems, and a similar number are lost because of industrial accidents which can be traced to stressful working conditions. Stress has also been thought to contribute to low job satisfaction, absenteeism, poor labour relations, high labour turnover and low productivity. The possible sources of stress at work can be divided into a number of categories.

Working conditions

● Excessive noise makes it hard to concentrate and to hear others speak. Prolonged high noise levels can lead to hearing loss.

● Movement and vibration can cause blurred vision and difficulty in performing co-ordinated movements. It can also cause nausea.

● Lower temperatures are required for physically demanding work than for sedentary office jobs because the exertion generates warmth. People vary a good deal in their preferred temperature for working.

The job itself

● Many occupations are very hazardous—for example: soldiers, divers and bomb disposal experts all regularly work under conditions of some danger. Not all such workers will perceive their work as particularly stressful because 'nervous' types will not go in for these occupations in the first place. Furthermore employers will try to avoid selecting obviously stress-prone applicants.

● Working long hours can be very stressful. One study suggested that men working more than 48 hours per week had double the risk of dying of heart disease of men working less than 40 hours. Another study looked at 100 young patients in hospital with heart disease. A quarter of them had been working at two jobs, and nearly half of them had been working more than 60 hours per week.

●Having to work at a very fast rate, especially for extended periods of

Below: *Much of the stress involved in being an airline pilot stems from the weight of responsibility—for up to 500 passengers and cabin crew on a big airliner.*

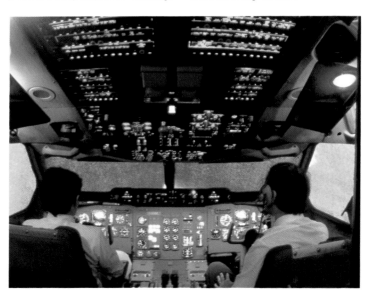

time, can be highly stressful. When the rate of work is governed by a machine, as in assembly-line conveyor-belt work, operators are particularly likely to report low job satisfaction and to develop stress-related illnesses. They are also prone to industrial accidents because they tend to 'switch off' mentally.

• Work overload is often a problem. This may be of two kinds: 'too much' or 'too difficult'. Too much work often goes together with long hours. Workers with too much to do tend to drink and smoke more than less overworked colleagues. In some cases work overload is not determined by the job itself but by the worker who, for various reasons, takes on too much. Too little work may also be a source of stress.

Role
• Stress may arise when the requirements of the job are unclear or ambiguous, or when different aspects of the job appear to conflict with each other.

• Responsibility is a powerful source of stress, particularly if it involves responsibility for other people. Bus drivers, ambulance staff and air traffic controllers are very prone to this. It also affects health care workers such as doctors, nurses and social workers, all of whom have responsibilities toward their patients and clients. Continuous stress of this nature can destroy the ability to cope with the demands of the job, a condition which has been called 'burnout'.

Relationships with others
If your relationships with superiors, subordinates, fellow workers or clients are marked by hostility, competitiveness or lack of appreciation, you are likely to find the job stressful. The situation when workers feel they are not involved in decision-making can have the same effect.

Job prospects
Your job future may be problematic in two different ways. The job itself may not be secure—that is, there may be a threat of premature

Below: *Danger is an obvious source of stress, but because the hazards are very apparent, such occupations generally only attract people who know they can cope.*

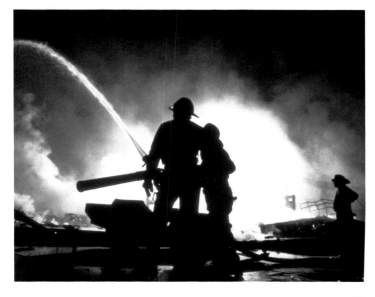

retirement or redundancy. Alternatively your chances of progress, development and promotion may be blocked. Both situations can cause stress, although it is likely to be much more acute in the face of redundancy.

Domestic conflict

In some marriages one partner, usually the husband, goes out to work. In others both partners work. The balance of their personalities and needs can determine whether the work experience of either is stressful or not. A typical combination is that of an ambitious, work-oriented husband and an unambitious, home-oriented wife. This can be a stable and happy arrangement in which the needs of both are met. In some marriages, however, the needs and wishes of each partner do not balance, leading to stress both at home and at work.

Stress at work may be better understood if we ask the question 'Why do we work? According to one influential theorist, Abraham Maslow, we all have five kinds of needs which should be met if we are to find our work fulfilling. At the lowest and most fundamental level, we have basic physiological needs, like food and water, which are necessary for life. At the next level

there is the need for safety and freedom from harm. The third level of need is for friendship. The fourth level consists of the need for self-esteem and respect and appreciation by others. At the highest level is a need for what Maslow called 'self-actualization'. This means the opportunity for personal growth and development and the expansion of one's abilities and horizons.

According to Maslow these five needs are arranged in a hierarchy with physiological needs at the bottom and self-actualization at the top. Low-level needs like physiological and safety requirements must be satisified before those higher in the hierarchy can be attended to.

At the most elementary level a job must provide sufficient rewards in terms of pay and fringe benefits, but ideally a job should satisfy a worker at all five levels. Maslow's model goes some way to explaining why jobs which provide a living wage may still be regarded as frustrating and stressful. A job may provide the basic necessities of life and be free from environmental hazards, but if

Below: *Maslow's hierarchy of human needs shows how basic requirements must be satisfied before higher ones can be met.*

MASLOW'S HIERARCHY OF HUMAN NEEDS

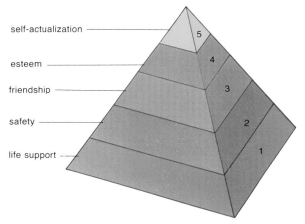

self-actualization — 5

esteem — 4

friendship — 3

safety — 2

life support — 1

JOB STRESS		
I get on well with my boss	YES	NO
I have too much or too little work to do	NO	YES
In my job one gets into trouble for making mistakes	NO	YES
I feel undervalued in my job	NO	YES
There are many time pressures and deadlines in my job	NO	YES
I get on well with my colleagues	YES	NO
My promotion prospects are good	YES	NO
My job pays reasonably well	YES	NO
My job affects my private life	NO	YES
My husband/wife has a positive attitude towards my work	YES	NO
I often take work home with me	NO	YES
I have responsibility for other people in my job	NO	YES
There is a lot of 'office politics' in my job	NO	YES
I don't have much opportunity to influence events in my job	NO	YES
My beliefs conflict with those of the firm I work for	NO	YES
I get on well with my subordinates	YES	NO
There is not much consultation or communication where I work	NO	YES
My job is well defined	YES	NO
There is conflict between my work group and others in the organization	NO	YES
The management doesn't understand my work problems	NO	YES

The more questions you answered in the right-hand column, the more stressful your job is to you. Some job stress is unavoidable, but if most of your answers indicate stress you should try to do something about it.

it cannot provide social stimulation, a sense of personal worth, and opportunities for bettering oneself and exploiting one's abilities to the full, it may yet be very low on job satisfaction and be a source of considerable stress.

Person-environment fit
One approach to the understanding of stress at work concerns the way the worker and the work environment fit together. This approach proposes that work stress arises not so much from the weaknesses or needs of the worker, nor from the excessive demands of the work environment, but from a mismatch between the two.

Four elements are involved. The

actual environment refers to the real demands of the job, whether these are formally specified by the employer or not. The perceived environment represents the worker's own perception of the demands of the job. This may be based upon what he has been told or has otherwise learned from his employer and workmates. The actual ability refers to the real skills of the worker, while the perceived ability represents his perception or opinion of his skills. These four

Below: The UK death rate from stress-related causes among various professions. These are standardized mortality ratios, i.e. 100 is the average for all workers.

OCCUPATIONAL STRESS				
	Coronary heart disease	Stroke	Duodenal ulcer	Suicide
Company directors	758	1925	485	700
Civil servants	118	446	107	125
Labourers	118	138	176	188
Ship's officers	152	111	110	125
Doctors	118	176	110	67
Miners	98	105	116	107
Clerical workers	119	107	99	94
Lawyers, judges	93	133	84	100
Gardeners	82	119	90	81
Farmers	69	84	71	117
Artists	96	85	58	94
Accountants	93	91	92	31
Administrators	95	73	50	63
Politicians	97	30	86	44
Clergymen	90	53	83	60

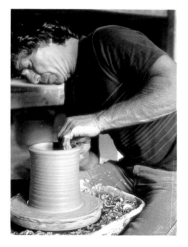

Above: *Work is not always a source of stress. If the job matches the worker, it can be very satisfying.* Below: *Person-environment misfit is a major source of work stress. This diagram shows the four main mismatches that can occur between the actual demands of the job and abilities of the worker, and the worker's perception of those demands and abilities.*

elements are all interconnected (see diagram) and for each interconnection a 'mismatch' means a potential problem.

When the perceived environment is inconsistent with the actual environment then the worker obviously has an inaccurate notion of the true requirements of the job. The worker may believe that the demands are greater or less than they really are. This kind of problem could be reduced by the provision of a clear, detailed job description.

A mismatch between actual ability and perceived ability implies a faulty perception on the worker's part of his or her own capabilities.

One form of misfit is between actual ability and the actual environment. This may be because the worker is underskilled (or perhaps overskilled) for the job — the consequence will be inefficiency. However, the clearest cause of work-related stress is the misfit between perceived environment and perceived ability, which represents the discrepancy between what the worker thinks is required by the job and what he thinks he is capable of.

PERSON-ENVIRONMENT FIT

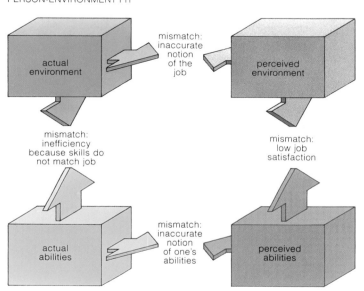

For many people the only thing more stressful than work is not being in work. At a time of world-wide economic recession the problem of unemployment has become an issue for society as a whole. There is now considerable evidence that unemployment and poor physical health are related — the unemployed appear to be more prone to a wide variety of illnesses. But does unemployment *cause* these illnesses? Could it be that the less fit members of the workforce are more likely to lose their jobs and less likely to be re-employed? This seems not to be the case. Studies have shown that periods of ill-health often start during unemployment, and a return to work often coincides with an improvement in health.

Although less obvious, one's psychological health can also be adversely affected by periods of unemployment. Strain and worry are most apparent in the first few months following job loss; after that a certain amount of readjustment and re-patterning of life often occurs, and the problems diminish.

Professor Peter Warr of the University of Sheffield has identified a number of stresses associated with unemployment:

• First, and most obvious, is money. Most unemployed people have drastically reduced incomes, and worry over financial commitments is a powerful stressor. Money worries may be more of a problem for the older unemployed who generally have greater financial commitments than the younger unemployed.

• For many, but not all, a job provides aims, ambitions and goals. The loss of the motivating effect supplied by work can lead to feelings of aimlessness which can become very stressful.

• For the unemployed, the variety and diversity of life is much reduced. Activities and interests are restricted, partly through lack of contact with workmates and partly through lack of money.

• Skills fall into disuse with unemployment. The long-term unemployed may become so rusty and 'de-skilled' that it becomes difficult to re-enter the job market when openings arise.

• One's sense of personal freedom is largely derived from the ability to make decisions, especially important decisions. Unemployment reduces options, narrows horizons and results in a reduced sense of personal choice.

• The social life of the jobless is often diminished. Even when unemployed people spend as much time socializing as formerly it is likely to be with a smaller circle of friends.

• The unemployed are likely to experience feelings of anxiety and insecurity in connection with the future. Many aspects of life which previously seemed secure, such as housing, come to look uncertain.

• Finally, one's personal sense of

Below: *Getting involved in some alternative work can help prevent the feelings of aimlessness and inferiority which often afflict the unemployed.*

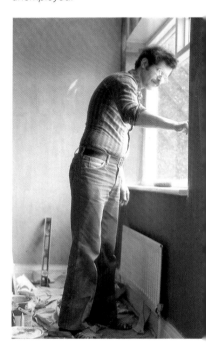

worth and self-esteem is vulnerable to the effects of unemployment. It is difficult for unemployed people to avoid feeling inferior and of less worth to society.

Just how stressful unemployment will be for any given person will depend on a number of factors. Clearly the extent to which someone *desires* work is important. Not surprisingly joblessness hits hardest those who want a job. A small but significant minority of people say they feel *better* for not having a job. There is some evidence that unemployment is more stressful for the middle-aged than it is for either school leavers, who are less likely to have financial commitments, or older people who would be anticipating retirement. Studies suggest that loss of a job may be more difficult to cope with

Below: *Like unemployment, retiring from regular work can make people lose direction and self-esteem. It is essential to take a positive view and enjoy it.*

for those who have been in blue collar work (skilled, semi-skilled and unskilled) than white collar (managerial and professional) workers. This is probably because ex-blue collar workers have more financial problems and a smaller range of alternative activities.

Coping with unemployment

A job gives structure to time, and in the absence of a job it is easy to drift into aimlessness and apathy. Establishing a regular daily and weekly routine will help prevent this happening. A sense of social worth may be recaptured either through partial work (a part-time job or job-sharing) or through voluntary or charitable activities. These will also widen social horizons and prevent the feeling of isolation which often affects the unemployed. Purpose and direction may be gained by self-improvement through educational and training courses. The development of satisfying 'leisure' pursuits also has an important role to play.

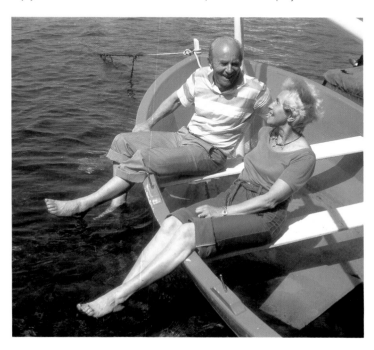

STRESS MANAGEMENT

There are many ways in which people can counteract the effects of stress and achieve a relaxed state of mind and body. Some of these methods involve the use of external agents, such as medicines, drugs and electronic devices, while others employ physical and mental techniques, such as relaxation training and meditation. A rather different approach involves trying to get rid of or modify the circumstances which are causing the stress, tension or anxiety in the first place.

Psychologists recognize that it is not always possible to avoid stressful conditions completely, and for this reason they talk of stress management rather than stress relief. When stress, anxiety or fear cannot be overcome completely it is always helpful to know that you can cope with or tolerate your stress reaction even if you can't get rid of it altogether.

All the methods which have been developed have their advantages and disadvantages. Medicines and other drugs, such as alcohol, are convenient, generally work quickly and can be quite powerful in their effects. But they can be expensive, habit-forming and become weaker in their effects if used for a long time. In addition, they give the user little future protection against stress symptoms.

Various instruments and gadgets, which are described further in the section on biofeedback (see page 66) can be very useful in helping to detect the signs of stress and in reducing it. Many of them are miniaturized and battery-operated, so they are particularly suitable for carrying around with you. One of their drawbacks is that they are often quite expensive.

Relaxation training and related techniques are excellent general-purpose ways of combating anxiety and tension. They lack all of the disadvantages of medicines but require a certain amount of time to learn and practice.

The removal or modification of stress-producing conditions is in

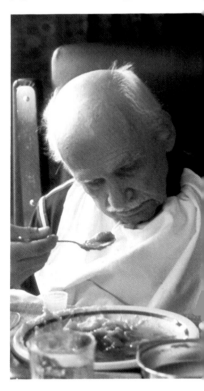

Above: *The stress involved in caring for a disabled relative cannot be avoided — but it can be controlled.* Right: *Learn how to relax!*

many ways the best remedy of all. Unfortunately this is not always possible. Sometimes individuals are subject to multiple sources of stress. In other cases, the stress-producing conditions cannot be easily removed — for example unemployment or caring for a sick relative.

No single stress management technique is the best. Some are more suitable for short-term crises which can be expected to be over soon, whilst others are more appropriate for stress reactions which last for some time. Individual preferences come into it too. A method which suits one person and is effective for him or her may have little to offer someone else.

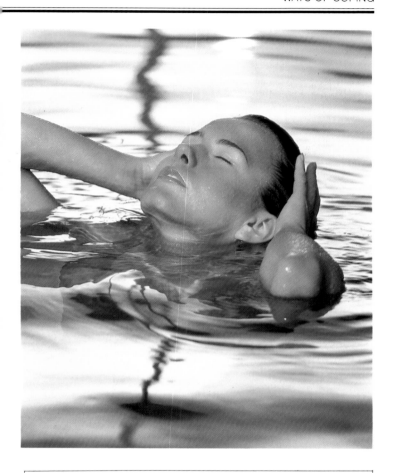

THE 'STRESS-PROOF' PERSONALITY

Some people have a personality characteristic known as 'hardiness' which helps protect them against the effects of stress. Hardiness consists of *commitment* to one's work, family or other important areas of life; *control,* or the belief that one can influence what happens in one's world; and *challenge*, or an eagerness for change and a constant flow of new experiences.

A study which compared the characteristics of both ill and healthy workers in one high-stress occupation showed that the healthy workers had much more of the three components of hardiness. This and other similar studies suggest that 'hardy' individuals are less likely to suffer physical or mental problems as a consequence of stress. They can keep events in perspective through their long-term commitments, they trust their personal coping resources, and they view potentially stressful developments as opportunities for change and growth.

Such people are lucky to be naturally stress-resistant. Less fortunate individuals have to work at it.

55

It is probably not too much of an overstatement to say that the most popular and widely-used method of overcoming the effects of stress is to swallow something. A famous physician once remarked that the main thing that distinguishes man from other animals is his desire to take drugs. All manner of such substances, some legal, some illegal, some solid (pills) some liquid (alcohol) are used for this purpose. Undoubtedly the main reason for the widespread use of substances for coping with stress is their effectiveness, their convenience and, in the case of medically prescribed drugs, the fact that they are believed in and recommended by the doctor who prescribes them.

Of course, drugs have their drawbacks as well. They are sometimes accused of treating the consequences of stress without tackling the cause. Some drugs

Below: *Quick and easy, drugs which combat stress symptoms such as anxiety and depression are among the most commonly prescribed of all medicines.*

Right: *A variety of drugs, both legal and illegal, are used to modify mental states. While effective, all have disadvantages; some are positively dangerous.*

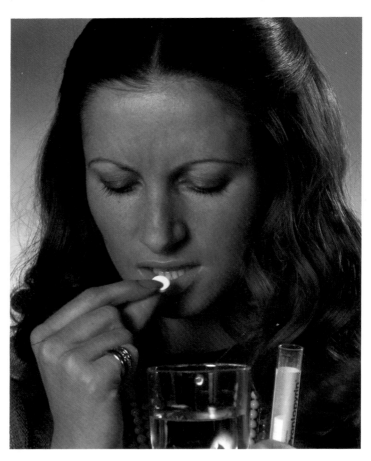

start to lose their chemical effect when they are taken continuously for a prolonged period of many months. Most anti-anxiety drugs have some side-effects, which can be undesirable and unpleasant. A few drugs, especially alcohol, are habit-forming and addictive, and the difficulties some people experience when trying to stop taking drugs after habits or addictions have been established can be worse than the problems the drugs were taken for in the first place. Finally, the anxiety-relieving properties of all drugs are only effective when just the right amount is taken—not too little and not too much. A few drugs are positively poisonous when too much is taken, or when they are taken in combination with another drug (commonly alcohol) which exaggerates their effects. Fortunately modern anxiety-reducing drugs have fewer of these

DRUGS WITH PSYCHOLOGICAL AND MENTAL EFFECTS

Drugs which suppress or inhibit or psychological processes or feelings	Drugs which stimulate or excite psychological processes or feelings	Drugs which produce abnormal psychological processes, perceptions or feelings
Major tranquillizers e.g. chlorpromazine (Largactil)	Anti-depressants e.g. imipramine (Tofranil)	LSD and related drugs
Minor tranquillizers e.g. diazepam (Valium)	Stimulants e.g. amphetamine caffeine	Cannabis
Sedatives e.g. alcohol		

Advantages	Disadvantages
Drugs have strong anxiety-reducing properties	Drugs will not get rid of the cause of the anxiety
Drugs are easy and convenient to use	Some drugs lose their effectiveness when taken for a long time
Most drugs work quickly	Some drugs have undesirable side-effects
Drugs are useful to deal with a short-term crisis	Some drugs are habit-forming
	Some drugs are poisonous when taken in excess

disadvantages than used to be the case some years ago.

A drug may be thought of as any substance which is taken into the body with the purpose of changing some body function or the way we feel. The list on page 57 gives the main classes of drugs which affect mood or mental state. By no means all of the drugs listed there are used against anxiety, tension or stress. The main groups which are used for that purpose are the minor tranquillizers, anti-depressants and alcohol.

Minor tranquillizers
This group of drugs is so called to distinguish them from the major tranquillizers which are employed in the treatment of the severer forms of mental illness and to subdue disturbed or violent behaviour. The best known minor tranquillizers are a chemical family called the benzodiazepines. Within this family there are diazepam (Valium), chlordiazepoxide (Librium), lorazepam (Ativan), oxazepam (Serenid), nitrazepam (Mogadon) and others. The names in brackets are the common brand names used worldwide.

The benzodiazepines are the most commonly prescribed group of drugs in the world, and diazepam (Valium) is the single most heavily prescribed drug. Benzodiazepines are popular because they are effective, non-poisonous and they have fewer and milder troublesome side-effects than other drugs given for similar problems. Nitrazepam (Mogadon) is well known as a sleeping pill, and it may seem a little surprising to see it in the same family as drugs which are used as tranquillizers. The fact is that all benzodiazepines when used in low doses have tranquillizing effects, and when used in high doses induce sleep. Overdoses with benzodiazepines alone usually result in little worse than a very long, very deep sleep.

Until quite recently it was thought that benzodiazepines were not addictive, but lately this belief has been proved wrong. People who suddenly stop taking their benzodiazepine medication after having used it continuously for a long time are likely to suffer a 'withdrawal' reaction. This may involve sweating, trembling, palpitations, anxiety, panic and peculiar feelings in various parts of

Right: *Drugs for short-term problems can become a habit.*

DID YOU KNOW?

● About 40 million tranquillizers are consumed each day by people all over the world.

● In Britain, between 1 in 40 and 1 in 50 of all adults takes a tranquillizer every day of the year, even though it is doubtful if there is any chemical effect beyond four to six months.

● About one adult in every seven takes a tranquillizer at some time in each year.

●Twice as many women as men take a tranquillizer or sleeping pill at some time in each year.

● In each year more mood-altering drugs are prescribed than any other kind of medicine.

● The three bestselling drugs in the USA are a tranquillizer, a blood pressure drug, and an ulcer medication.

the body — in fact many of the feelings for which the drugs were prescribed for in the first place! Very occasionally convulsions (fits) may occur. The moral is, if you are taking benzodiazepines regularly, and want to give up, seek the help and guidance of your doctor and lower the dose gradually.

In spite of the excellent anti-anxiety properties of the common benzodiazepines, two other problems associated with their use need to be mentioned. One is that they do tend to affect alertness and judgement. This can make driving and operating heavy machinery hazardous. The other is the problem of reduced effectiveness. After four to six months of continuous use, the main benefits of these drugs are probably psychological rather than chemical.

Anti-depressants
When stress leads to depression, anti-depressant drugs may be prescribed. Of the various drugs which have been used to try to relieve depression, amphetamines such as dexedrine and methedrine are no longer employed because

they are highly addictive and can have a number of very unpleasant side-effects.

The recognized modern anti-depressants are the tricyclics, of which the most widely used are amitriptyline and imipramine (Tofranil); tetracyclics, notably mianserin (Bolvidon) and maprotiline (Ludiomil); and monoamine oxidase inhibitors (MAOIs) such as phenelzine (Nardil) and isocarboxazid (Marplan). The monamine oxidase inhibitors are less widely used than the other two groups, mainly because of their more troublesome side-effects and the need for dietary restrictions.

Both tranquillizers and anti-depressants have their place in the management of the most severe and distressing reactions to stress. In particular, they can be helpful in enabling people to 'get over the worst of it'. Modern medical opinion favours trying to limit the prescription of these drugs to shortish intervals, such as a couple of weeks or months, and to avoid using them continuously for many months or even years.

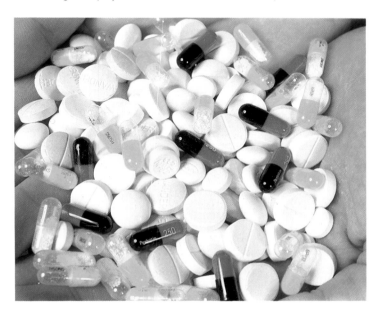

When we speak of relaxation as a means of coping with stress, we mean specific, systematic procedures for achieving physical and mental relaxation, not merely leisure or generally taking it easy. There are a number of relaxation methods; most of them concentrate on two techniques—breathing control and the regulation of muscular tension.

Stress and anxiety are often associated with muscular tension. This can be seen in a tense, pinched or frowning face and in a hunched or rigid posture. Any muscle which is activated for a long time will begin to tire, so generalized tension and anxiety often leads to stiffness, fatigue, and muscular aches and pains, especially around the shoulders, neck and head. We have two kinds of muscles in our bodies: the voluntary muscles and the involuntary muscles. The involuntary muscles are those over which we have no direct control, such as the muscles of our stomach

or our heart. The activity of these muscles is controlled mainly by the autonomic nervous system (see page 20). The voluntary muscles are those which we use for purposeful activity. It is these muscles—there are about 620 in the human body—which respond to relaxation techniques.

Breathing control is the other major component of relaxation training. Breathing and muscular tension are quite closely connected. Our muscles tend to tense up when we breathe in and relax again when we breathe out. Stretching and yawning (tensing the muscles and breathing in deeply) is an example of this.

Relaxation training is a self-control method which harnesses

Right: *The effect of massage is physical and psychological—it is pleasant to be pampered.*
Below: *Autogenic training uses the power of the imagination to induce a relaxed state.*

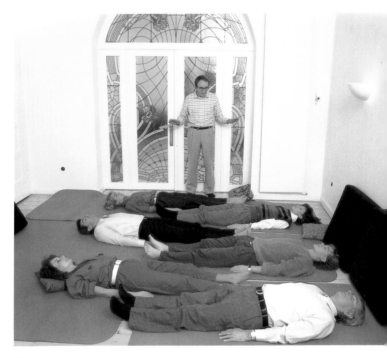

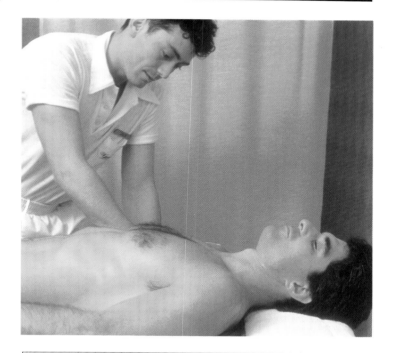

MASSAGE

Massage helps relax the muscles, and creates a general feeling of well-being. We all know that rubbing a painful spot can help dispel pain. Athletes often have a rub-down after strenuous physical exertion to counteract the aching of tired limbs. Physiologically, massage increases the blood flow through the muscles which enables the waste products generated by muscular activity to be carried away more rapidly. In addition to these actual physical effects, the pleasurable sensations from skin contact and stroking help dispel psychological tension. Massage of certain key areas, such as the shoulders, neck and back, will promote muscular and general relaxation. Remember, everyone likes to feel kneaded.

AUTOGENIC TRAINING

Autogenic training is a relaxation technique which does not involve muscular activity or physical contact. It is a method which works through imagination and auto-suggestion.

Adopting a reclining position with your eyes closed, turn your attention to each part of the body in turn and repeat to yourself the statement that it feels *heavy*: 'My right leg feels heavy'. After working your way through the body in this way, go through them again with statements that they feel *warm*: 'My right leg feels warm'. After this, make self-statements to the effect that your *breathing* is calm and easy. Further, more specific self-statements may be added. Even though it is common to feel no direct sensations of heaviness or warmth, the procedure can be a very effective way of attaining a relaxed state.

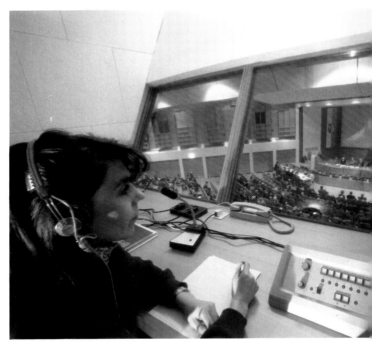

muscle contractions and breathing patterns to produce a state of physical and mental calmness.

Progressive muscular relaxation

This is a technique developed by Dr Edmund Jacobson of the University of Chicago in the 1930s. Before starting you require a quiet environment, free of distractions and noise, and a comfortable lying or reclining position. Begin by setting up a slow, deep and rhythmic pattern of breathing. This is the opposite of the fast, shallow and irregular breathing typical of anxiety and panic states. A momentary pause between breaths is helpful in slowing the breathing rate down and establishing a regular rhythm. Counting or saying 'in . . . out' to yourself can also be useful. A further point is the balance between the in-breath and the out-breath. During anxiety and panic the in-breath is usually longer than the out-breath, but when

Above: *People in high-pressure occupations, like this interpreter, can keep stress under control by regular use of relaxation methods.*

relaxed they are about equal or even the other way round. It is of overriding importance that the breathing be natural and unforced. With practice it can become so, and the pay-off in terms of relaxation is well worth it.

Once the correct breathing pattern is established, you can move on to contracting and relaxing the main muscle groups. You may wonder why it is that in order to get relaxed one needs to tense the muscles. There are two reasons. First, it enables the individual who is tense most or all of the time to become aware of the difference between a state of tension and a state of relaxation. Second, it has been found that relaxing a muscle immediately after having tensed it leads to a greater degree of muscle relaxation.

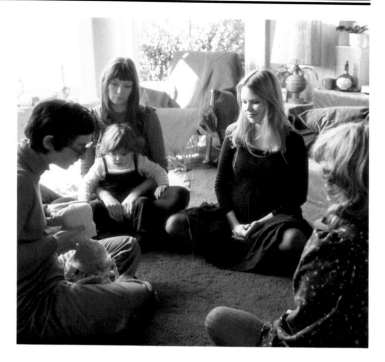

Above: *Relaxation techniques have very wide application, and are taught in ante-natal classes to ease the pain of childbirth.*

In progressive muscular relaxation the major muscle groups in the body are tensed and relaxed in sequence: feet, calves, thighs, buttocks, abdomen, chest, shoulders, arms, hands, neck, head and face. In each case the muscles are tensed up on the in-breath and relaxed on the out-breath. If one part is rather more difficult to relax than the others the process may be repeated one or more times. The whole process should be natural and pleasurable, and it need not take a long time. A typical relaxation session may last ten to twenty minutes. Two such sessions a day are considered ideal for most people.

Sometimes busy people who live hectic lives, who could benefit from relaxation training ask 'How can I find the time and the circumstances to do systematic relaxation regularly? In fact the time requirements for progressive muscular relaxation are very modest, and one relaxation session in the evening after work is usually possible for everyone.

Relaxation has proved its worth as a remedy for all kinds of problems and in all kinds of situations. The limbering-up exercises practised by athletes, musicians and others preparing for highly co-ordinated activity are related to relaxation techniques, and certainly help to calm the nerves. Antenatal classes for mothers-to-be make childbirth itself easier and less painful by relaxing the muscles. Relaxation before and during a visit to the dentist will reduce stress and can reduce the pain of drilling and injections. Furthermore, although relaxation when done properly should leave one feeling alert and not at all sleepy, it has been used very successfully to combat sleeplessness.

Meditation, which takes several different forms and styles, means the achievement of a state of mental stillness by focussing the mind on a single object or idea. The best known forms of meditation, like Zen and Transcendental Meditation, derive originally from the religions and philosophies of the East, but it is possible to find meditational approaches originating from the West too: Christian mystics and teachers, like St Augustine and St Teresa, were aware of the connection between meditation and prayer.

It is widely held that there are four main elements of meditation. First, it is necessary to have a quiet environment. This is essential if you are not to be distracted by sights and sounds. Second, you need a comfortable position. The positions usually adopted by meditators are either sitting or kneeling, but in general, any comfortable position in which the spine is straight is satisfactory. Some of the positions involving twisted limbs adopted by Yoga meditators seem far from comfortable, and cannot be recommended for beginners. The important point about all meditational postures is that once achieved they can be maintained without additional muscular effort. Third, you need to adopt a passive attitude, that is to say, suspend your judgement and critical faculties and allow the meditational process to take over. These three elements are also essential to relaxation training (see page 60), but the fourth, concentrating on a single object or idea, is distinctive to meditation. Many objects or ideas have been used for the purposes of meditation: a candle flame, a single word like 'love' or 'peace', or an object with religious or symbolic significance, such as a cross. In Transcendental Meditation word or sound called a mantra is given to each meditator. The rhythmic repetition of the mantra is then an essential part of the meditational process.

Experiments have shown that during meditation the metabolism, which is the rate at which the body burns up energy, decreases. So does oxygen consumption, heart rate and blood lactate (the level of lactate in the blood is high during episodes of anxiety and panic). Highly-skilled meditators can get their heart rate down to three or four beats per minute, and meditational approaches have been successfully used to treat high blood pressure. The meditational state has been likened in its physical effects to sleep and hibernation, but there are important differences. Unlike the sleeper the meditator is fully alert and unlike the hibernating animal the meditator's temperature does not fall, indeed, experienced meditators report greater alertness and improved concentration in addition to the benefits of relaxation.

Meditation is a relatively simple,

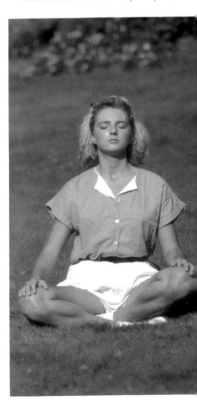

TRANSCENDENTAL MEDITATION

This is a very useful technique, which can be employed anytime, anywhere—even on the train going to work. All you need is a quiet place where you will be undisturbed for 15 minutes, and a mantra: a soothing word such as 'sun' which is silently repeated over and over again. There is no need to adopt an exotic yoga position; simply sitting in a comfortable chair that supports your back is ideal.

• Sit quietly, close your eyes, and relax.

• Begin repeating to yourself the word you have chosen as a mantra: 'sun ... sun ... sun ...'

• Whenever you are distracted, or your attention wanders, gently turn your mind back to repeating the mantra.

• Keep the repetition going for 15 minutes or more. You will find that it clears your brain of all the mental clutter that has built up, and helps to free you from anxiety.

• Finally, stop the repetition, but remain sitting calmly. Open your eyes.

Left: *Meditation needs a soothing, quiet environment: the garden in summer is ideal, but a long train journey can also be used.*
Below: *During periods of inactivity the body needs less oxygen, indicating a reduction in stress. This effect is more marked during deep relaxation, and is most evident during meditation.*

straightforward way of dealing with stress. A single session generally occupies about twenty minutes, and two such sessions per day is considered sufficient for most people. The technique can be employed at just about any time of day, but it is not recommended immediately after meals or just before going to sleep.

THE PHYSICAL EFFECT OF MEDITATION

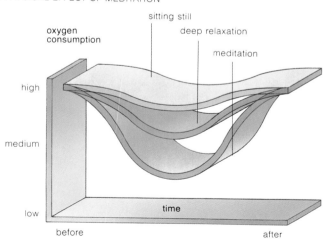

Biofeedback involves the use of instruments to measure certain physiological functions. These measurements are monitored by the user, who attempts to increase or decrease the level of activation to a more 'healthy' level by modifying his or her mental state. It has been found that, using this technique, people are able to achieve a degree of control over reactions and functions which are usually thought to be outside our control. Because of this, when a certain physical function such as muscle tension or heart rate reaches an abnormally high or abnormally low pitch as a result of stress, the biofeedback technique can be helpful in readjusting it to a healthy level.

One of the most widely practised forms of biofeedback involves the galvanic skin response. When we are tense or anxious we tend to sweat, and when we are relaxed our skin tends to be dry. When the skin is damp an electric current will pass more easily over it than when it is dry, because sweat is a good conductor of electricity. By placing electrodes on convenient points on the skin, such as the fingers, it is possible to measure the skin's electrical resistance: high when the skin is dry and low when its damp.

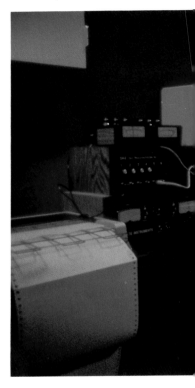

Above: *Biofeedback devices range from simple gadgets to multi-function monitors.*

THE LIE DETECTOR

A lie detector registers some of the physiological functions which are employed in biofeedback. In the lie detector test, however, several measures are taken simultaneously, rather than one as in normal biofeedback, and also the information is not relayed to the subject. Sudden changes in the monitored functions immediately after certain questions or answers indicate a change in the subject's level of arousal, or stress, and alert the examiner to the possibility that the answer is not truthful. The graph below shows the effect of a change in galvanic skin response which might be associated with a lie. This appears as a peak on the readout.

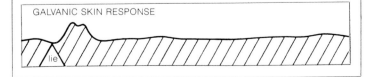

GALVANIC SKIN RESPONSE

lie

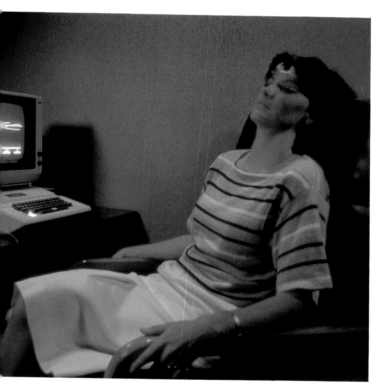

This information is usually conveyed to the subject in the form of a continuous tone of variable pitch: high-pitched when the skin is sweaty and low-pitched when it is dry. the task of the subject is to make the pitch of the tone go down and stay down, by somehow reducing his or her level of tension or anxiety.

The same basic approach can be used to feed back other physical states. The tension level of the muscles in the forehead can be fed back to people suffering from tension headaches, who can then try to reduce it. Biofeedback of muscle tension elsewhere in the body has been used in the treatment of involuntary muscle twinges, or tics. Electrodes on the scalp can detect electrical brain activity (alpha waves) which is present when one is relaxed but absent when one is aroused and alert. This system has been used for successful biofeedback treatment of sleeplessness. Blood pressure and heart rate biofeedback can be helpful to people with disorders of the circulatory system, whether these disorders are stress-related or not.

The instruments which are in biofeedback are extremely sensitive. Because of this only very small amounts of electricity need be used, and so the techniques are entirely safe. The small changes in electrical resistance are amplified and relayed back to the individual either as a tone or visually, as a pointer on a dial or as a trace on paper. Normally of course, we do not feel we have any control over such things as perspiration and heart rate, but it has been shown that with a trial-and-error approach, and persistence and practice, most people can gain some control.

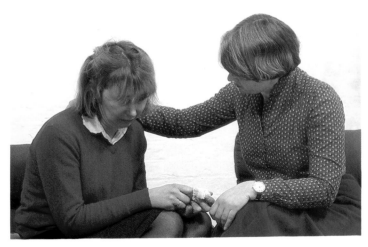

Above: A good counsellor must be able to establish a close, confiding and open relationship with the client.

Friendship, support and humane concern have always been recognized as beneficial to people under stress. Psychotherapy and counselling are forms of help for people with emotional difficulties which are provided by professional helpers, using the therapeutic power of the helping relationship.

Psychotherapy

Psychotherapy has been defined as a medium to long-term relationship between one participant (the patient) who has entered into it because he is dissatisfied with his emotional adjustment, and the other participant (the psychotherapist) who is a trained professional. The aim is the resolution of those difficulties for which the patient sought help, using methods which are psychological and interpersonal in nature.

The professional always operates according to a theory which explains the emotional disturbance and prescribes an appropriate therapy which will correct it. Psychotherapy in the modern sense has its origins with Anton Mesmer, the eighteenth-century hypnotist, who showed that he could abolish the symptoms of certain patients by putting them into a trance—an extreme form of therapy which is also a dramatic demonstration of the power of the doctor-patient relationship. Many theories and 'schools' of psychotherapy now exist; most of them originated from the ideas of Sigmund Freud, the founder of psychoanalysis, and his European colleagues.

All psychotherapies share certain common ingredients. The most important of these is a strong 'therapeutic alliance', which means a commitment by both parties to understanding and helping the client with his problems. It is essential that the therapist is a 'good listener'. Being a good listener involves more than just being a passive recipient of what the client has to say. It implies compassionate concern on the part of the therapist, who has to make a real effort to understand the personal meaning of the client's experiences. It is also important that the therapist respects the client's integrity, and acknowledges the individual nature of his problems. The basis of psychotherapy is talk. The therapist spends most of the time listening, asking questions, clarifying statements, exposing contradictions and explaining the meaning of the client's experiences and behaviour. The aim is to improve the client's understanding of himself and, in so doing reduce his difficulties.

Counselling

Stemming from an American rather than a European tradition, counselling operates at a simpler and less psychologically 'deep' level. The best-known writer on counselling, Carl Rogers, characterized the qualities of the ideal counsellor as genuineness, non-possessive warmth and accurate empathy. By genuineness he meant that a good counsellor is authentic and non-defensive in his behaviour. He does not hide behind a professional facade. Non-possessive warmth refers to the ability to establish a safe, non-threatening and trusting relationship in which the client is valued as an individual. Accurate empathy means the capacity to grasp the personal and emotional meaning of what the client says. For a person under stress, the opportunity to talk to someone who possesses these qualities is invaluable.

Although counselling and psychotherapy have been described here as they are practised by professionals, this is not to deny that the properties of a good professional relationship are comparable to the properties of any good helping relationship. The therapy provided by professionals has much in common with the help which can be provided by caring relatives and friends.

Those who stand to gain the most from psychotherapy and counselling as specific anti-stress techniques are people who are capable of seeing their symptoms, in particular their physical symptoms, as having a psychological basis, and who are willing and able to explore their own states of mind. Motivation is very important. Success will depend upon the patient's trust and willingness to participate in the therapeutic alliance, willingness to change and to experiment, and wish to understand himself better.

DEFINITIONS

Psychiatry
This is a branch of medicine concerned with the treatment of mental illness. Psychiatrists are medical doctors who are qualified to use a wide range of treatments including the prescription of medication.

Psychology
Psychology is the study of human behaviour and experience. Clinical psychologists are specialists in the treatment of emotional and behavioural problems by a variety of means, which do not involve medicines or drugs.

Psychotherapy
This term refers to the treatment of emotional problems by talk and thought. Psychotherapists are specially trained in these methods. Some psychotherapists are also trained in psychology or psychiatry, and vice versa.

Psychoanalysis
This is a system of psychotherapy derived from the work and ideas of Sigmund Freud and his colleagues and followers. The client's problems are traced back to his unconscious beliefs. In theory, once these are brought to light the problems tend to subside.

About 2000 years ago the Greek philosopher Epictetus said 'Men are disturbed not by things but by the views they take of them'. Rather more recently, Shakespeare had Hamlet saying 'there is nothing either good or bad, but thinking makes it so'. Cognitive methods are based upon the idea that it is our perception and evaluation—or cognition—of events that determine emotional upset and distress.

Psychologists working with people in emotional difficulties have been able to identify a number of *cognitive distortions,* by which they mean typical ways in which their clients misinterpret their experiences. These errors of thinking then lead them to draw unjustified conclusions about themselves; for example: that they are stupid, worthless, irresponsible or incompetent.

Closely connected with these cognitive distortions is the tendency for people to act and think according to internal 'rules' which demand an impossibly high standard of behaviour. Usually these rules are not spelled out in any way, but they can be inferred from the way people talk about themselves, their behaviour and events in their lives. Like all rules, they are expressed as 'musts' and 'shoulds'. The following are typical:
• I should never feel anxious. I must always be happy and calm.
• All hardships are to be endured no matter how difficult that may be.
• I should be able to understand and anticipate anything that may happen.
• I should always be in control of my feelings, but I should always be spontaneous too.
• I should assert myself but I should never hurt anyone's feelings.
• I should never be ill.
• It is wrong to have fun.
• I should be able to solve all my problems by myself.
• I should be a perfect husband/ wife/parent/citizen etc.

Cognitive treatments (also called cognitive restructuring) are designed to help the client identify

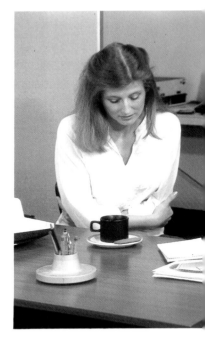

Above: *The stress of actual physical illness can be made worse by the belief that you never should be ill.*

his or her own self-defeating rules, and then enable the substitution of healthier or more realistic cognitions in their place.

There are three approaches: The 'intellectual' approach involves reasoning and debate between the client and therapist to test the validity of the client's cognitions. The 'experiential' approach relies on engaging the client in intense emotional experiences in order to challenge his misconceptions. Group work can be very effective at providing what has been called the 'corrective emotional experience'. The 'behavioural' approach involves directly modifying the client's behaviour patterns. It can be shown that altering behaviour can influence attitudes and self-perceptions, as well as vice versa.

Whichever avenue or combination of avenues is chosen

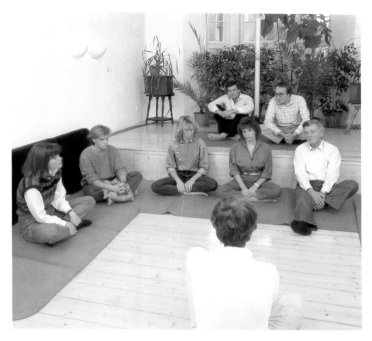

Above: *Group discussion is one way to create the emotional atmosphere which brings out deep-rooted misconceptions.*

the aim is to challenge the client's cognitions in a way that makes it practicable to modify or replace them. These methods are likely to work best with clients who are able and willing to be introspective and reflective.

Rational Emotive Therapy

The system of Rational Emotive Therapy, or RET, is an example of an 'intellectual' approach to stress problems. It can be conveniently summarized into five stages represented by the letters A,B,C,D and E. The letter A stands for the activating event — usually unpleasant — which is the source of the stress. For most people this stage appears to be followed immediately by stage C, the consequence: some form of emotional reaction. The use of the terms A and C makes it obvious that

a step has been missed out, and it is this in-between stage B, the belief, which is the real cause of the emotional reaction.

For example, the basic nature of an activating event such as retirement may be the same for two workers, but for one the consequence may be worry and apprehension while for the other it may be eager anticipation. The difference between them lies in their beliefs concerning the event: the first may believe that he is being written off as of no further use to his employers and to society, while the second may be looking forward to relief from a monotonous and tiring job. This difference in perception — the nature of their belief, or stage B — makes an enormous difference to the emotional reaction, or consequence (C), which is experienced by the two retiring workers. In RET, helping the client to understand that the apparent A-C sequence is in fact A-B-C is an important and necessary first stage in treatment.

COMMON COGNITIVE DISTORTIONS

'Black and white' thinking
Also known as dichotomous or polarized thinking, this means judging events in extreme terms. Sometimes this can be seen in a person's attitude to a failed exam or interview when he says (or thinks) 'I'm totally stupid' or 'nobody would want to employ me'. This implies that one is either a total success or a total failure. A more realistic assessment might be 'you win a few, you lose a few'.

Magnification
It is easy to place excessive importance on one event. An example is the person who acquires a slight blemish yet believes that he is badly disfigured. 'Catastrophizing' is an extreme form of magnification, in which every minor setback is seen as a disaster.

Minimization
Playing down the importance of an event or of some personal achievement is a common type of distorted thinking. A depressed doctor may dismiss the valuable treatment work he has done as insignificant. A depressed housewife may think she is worthless despite the important work she is doing in raising her children.

Personalization
Personalizing a situation means thinking that events are somehow connected with yourself when there is no good evidence for the belief. This may take the form of unwarranted feelings of guilt or responsibility. Personalisation is often seen in soldiers who have survived battles in which their friends have been killed.

Selective abstraction
This means basing your judgement on a small detail while ignoring the wider issue. This, along with magnification, is what people often mean when they talk about 'getting things out of proportion'.

Arbitrary inference
This means jumping to conclusions on the basis of insufficient, absent or even contrary evidence.

Overgeneralization
It is a common mistake to form rules or generalizations on the basis of one or a few isolated examples. In this way a person may feel, on the basis of a single failure, that he or she never does anything right.

The letter D refers to a number of related activities which are part of the treatment: debating, defining, disputing and distancing. These are part of a verbal process during which the client analyzes his beliefs and tests their validity, with the help of the therapist. Stage E, the final step in the sequence, stands for the effect of the whole undertaking, which should be a more mature, rational and objective outlook on life.

Top right: *A retirement party can be fun, but for some the prospect is simply depressing, because they believe they are being written off. Challenging such beliefs is an important part of stress therapy.* Right: *Cognitive distortions such as 'black and white' thinking can cause people to become quite despondent following setbacks. Awareness of such distortions will help in avoiding them.*

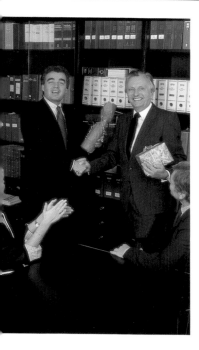

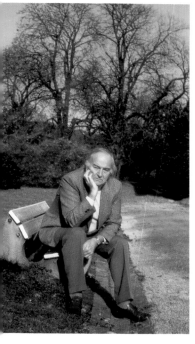

Stress Inoculation Training

Another system of teaching people how to cope with stress is known as Stress Inoculation Training. This is a three-part process, which begins with an educational phase in which the effects of stress on body functions, emotions and behaviour are explained to the client.

The second phase involves the rehearsal of coping techniques. The client is given relaxation training, and is also taught to mentally repeat a variety of statements which help to reduce stress reactions. These 'coping self-statements' then take the place of the negative self-statements which tend to be habitual with stress sufferers. Different coping self-statements are required at different stages of an anxiety-provoking event. In the period leading up to the event the client might be instructed to think 'recalling what I *can* do is better than getting anxious about what I *can't*'. One useful self-statement when handling or confronting the situation might be 'relax, and take a deep breath'. At the point when the client feels he may be overcome by panic, a self-statement such as 'this will be over soon' or 'think about something else' will be helpful. Once the crisis point has passed a self-statement like 'it wasn't as bad as I expected it to be' will improve the ability to cope with similar events in the future.

The third phase of Stress Inoculation Training involves practising these coping techniques in deliberately contrived stressful situations. Painful electric shocks, which can be adjusted for for severity and predictability, have been used for this purpose.

The Stress Inoculation Training package, comprising education, rehearsal and practice, has two particular strengths. First it enables the client to develop a sense of control over stressful situations. Second, as the term inoculation implies, it provides protection against a wide range of such situations in the future.

Over the decades the amount of time people spend at work has gradually declined. The normal working week is shorter, holiday entitlements have increased, and people retire earlier. Periods of temporary or prolonged unemployment are also increasingly common. In addition to this, labour-saving devices such as washing machines and food processors have drastically reduced the amount of time spent on domestic chores. The result is that the average person has a great deal of spare time.

The question of how to use spare time has become a major problem confronting developed societies. Education and training is largely geared to productive and economic use of time. Most of us are quite ill-equipped to use the free time made available to us by mechanization, automation and 'progress', and find it very difficult to relax.

Despite this it is clear that the value of leisure lies in the opportunity to relax and recover from the stresses and strains of everyday life. Everyone needs a certain amount of recreation, whether it takes the form of mental diversion and stimulation, or physical activity such as a sport. The word 'recreation', after all, means the refreshment of the spirit and the recharging of one's batteries. Leisure activities need not be frivolous and pointless; spare time may be equally well spent on valuable and 'serious' pursuits such as further education, or involvement with charitable and voluntary organisations. As long as the associated level of anxiety is low, such activities are equally effective as forms of recreation.

The person who needs to pay greatest attention to the use of his leisure time is the compulsive worker—the 'workaholic'. This is the individual who voluntarily works very long hours, works quickly and may be—but is not always—super-efficient. Typically he hates holidays, dreads retirement and fears boredom and inactivity. In many ways he corresponds to the 'Type A' personality described on page 30. Wise use of leisure time may well serve to lengthen the lifespan of this kind of person. Employers have their part to play by providing leisure facilities and by ensuring that employees work sensible hours and take the holidays they are entitled to.

Physical exercise

Regular physical exercise is an important weapon in the campaign against stress. Apart from the mental diversion it provides, the resulting improvement in physical fitness will help to counteract the physiological effects of anxiety. Use

Below: *An absorbing hobby provides valuable distraction from everyday stresses—but it is important to avoid anything which is too demanding.*

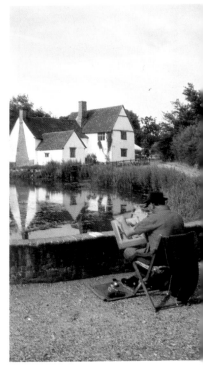

caution, though. If you are not particularly fit, or not used to strenuous physical exercise, the golden rule is 'start slowly and progress gradually'. If you experience unexpected pains, breathlessness or distress consult your doctor before proceeding. Exercise need not be especially strenuous to be effective at relieving stress—many people find simply walking very relaxing.

Non-team sports such as walking, running, swimming, and golf are generally preferable to intensely competitive team games like football. This is because there is a hard, aggressive edge to many team games which can be stressful in its own right. Also, each player

Below: Physical exercise in the open air is one of the best forms of stress therapy, provided it does not encourage any stress-provoking competitiveness.

has a responsibility to the whole team and the burden of this responsibility can be experienced as a stressful pressure.

Hobbies
There are many relaxing pastimes and leisure pursuits which do not involve physical exercise. Everyone should try to develop an interest in one or more of these, if only because the weather, physical injury, illness or old age may render sport impossible. As with sports and exercise, the most stress-relieving pursuits are those which are solitary and non-competitive, such as gardening, fishing, painting and reading. Ideally such pastimes should be interesting and mentally stimulating, without demanding a high level of skill, for this could lead to frustration. Activities which require excessive time commitments or involve competition against others are best avoided.

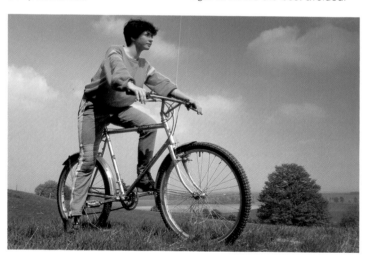

PET THERAPY
Pets can play a very useful part in the campaign against stress. For people living on their own, who might otherwise feel lonely, aimless and isolated, they provide much-needed company, a sense of responsibility and a certain amount of exercise. Indeed, research has shown that lonely heart attack victims with pets tend to live longer than those who do not have pets.

INDEX

PICTURE CREDITS

Artists Copyright of the artwork illustrations on the pages following the artists' names is the property of Salamander Books Ltd.
Milne Stebbing Illustration: 8, 9, 17, 21, 28, 33, 36, 37, 43, 48, 51, 65

Photographers The publishers wish to thank the following photographers and agencies who have supplied photographs for this book. The photographs have been credited by page number and position on the page where appropriate: (B) bottom, (T) top, (BL) bottom left etc.
Image Bank: (Gary Crallé) 5, (Kay Chernush) 12, (Alfred Gescheidt) 34, (R. Miguel) 61, (Zao-Longfield) 64, (Marc St Gil) 66-7
Kobal Collection: 18-19
Richard Revels: 38
Zefa: 6, 8, 10, 13, 22, 23, 24, 25, 26, 27, 29, 30(T), 30(B), 32, 39, 40, 41, 42(B), 45, 46, 47, 51, 52, 53, 54, 56, 59, 60, 62, 63, 68, 70, 71, 73(T), 73(B), back cover.

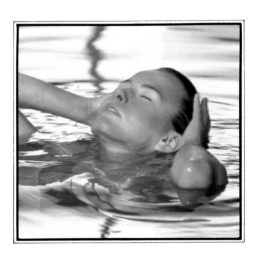